Consumer's Guide to FREE Medical INFORMATION by Phone and by Mail

ARTHUR WINTER, M.D., F.I.C.S.
AND RUTH WINTER, M.S.

PRENTICE HALL
Englewood Cliffs, New Jersey 07632

Prentice-Hall International (UK) Limited, *London*
Prentice-Hall of Australia Pty. Limited, *Sydney*
Prentice-Hall Canada, Inc., *Toronto*
Prentice-Hall Hispanoamericana, S.A., *Mexico*
Prentice-Hall of India Private Limited, *New Delhi*
Prentice-Hall of Japan, Inc., *Tokyo*
Simon & Schuster Asia Pte. Ltd., *Singapore*
Editora Prentice-Hall do Brasil, Ltda., *Rio de Janeiro*

10 9 8 7 6 5 4 3 2 1

Library of Congress Cataloging-in-Publication Data

Winter, Ruth
Consumer's guide to free medical information by phone and by mail/ by Ruth Winter and Arthur Winter.
p. cm.
ISBN 0-13-096199-X ISBN 0-13-333535-6
1. Medicine—Information services—United States—Directories. 2. Consumer education. I. Winter, Arthur. II. Title.
R118.4.U6W56 1993 92-24402
610—dc20 CIP

ISBN 0-13-096199-X

ISBN 0-13-333535-6 (P)

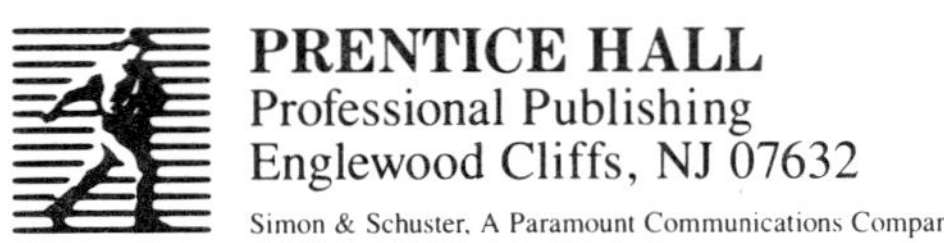

Printed in the United States of America

INTRODUCTION

Free medical information is available on almost every health condition and health-related topic from AIDS, aging, and cholesterol to diabetes, headaches, and weight loss. But finding the sources for this information can be a long and difficult process. *Consumer's Guide to Free Medical Information by Phone and by Mail* will provide you with easy access to accurate, up-to-date information on 315 key health topics, ranging from sports injuries to the latest new treatments for cancer.

This unique, all-in-one resource includes descriptions of *over 400* organizations and institutions that offer free medical information and assistance—medical, emotional, and sometimes financial—by phone and/or by mail. Many provide 800 number hotlines. Among the groups included in the book are federal and state agencies, medical schools, and organizations with specific health concerns such as the American Heart Association and the American Cancer Society. At your request, many of these organizations will refer you to medical experts and support groups located in your area.

All the groups listed filled out questionnaires designed especially for this book to ensure that the information presented would be as accurate, up to date, and comprehensive as possible.

HOW TO USE THIS BOOK

For easy use, the *Guide* is organized alphabetically by subject heading. Each subject heading is followed by a brief introduction to the topic and then by the specific listings. Provided for each listing are

- A detailed description of the group or organization
- The aim/purpose of the group or organization
- Publications available
- Special services offered
- Current address and phone number
- A toll-free 800 hotline number, if available.

While most organizations have toll-free 800 numbers, we have also given you office numbers, when possible, because you may be in a hurry to obtain the information you need, and 800 numbers can sometimes be endlessly busy. Furthermore, during nonbusiness hours or as a policy, you may get recorded messages on the 800 numbers or be requested to leave your name and number for a return call.

The printed material and the videotapes listed are free, but some of the groups also offer other useful materials for sale.

Please be patient when dealing with requests by mail. Some government agencies take as long as five weeks to send information. All organizations are active and at the locations noted as this book is being developed. If you are unable to obtain the information by phone or mail as described in the book, or you are a member of an organization that should be listed and is not, please let us know by sending a postcard to New Jersey Neurological Institute, 22 Old Short Hills Road, Short Hills, New Jersey 07039.

A Final Note

We wrote this book to help you gain the knowledge you need to ask the right medical questions and know where and how to obtain the best health care and comfort possible, no matter what ails you or your loved ones. The information you acquire will ease your anxiety and give you a sense of control over an illness or a situation that may have made you feel helpless. Francis Bacon summed it up when he said, "Knowledge is power." Armed with the medical knowledge available from the sources in this book, you can become an active participant in your own health care and the health care of those you love.

But, remember, this book is not a substitute for your doctor, and a listing in the book does not, in any way, guarantee that the information provided is correct, not even from government agencies or leading health organizations. This *Guide* is a means by which you can gather as much "intelligence" as you can about a health subject that is of interest or concern to you. It is up to you to ask pertinent questions, provide a complete medical history, and finally make your own informed choices.

We hope this book will help you make the best and most intelligent choices possible. Your life or the lives of your loved ones may depend upon it.

Arthur Winter, M.D., F.I.C.S.
Director, New Jersey Neurological Institute

Ruth Winter, M.S.
Livingston, NJ 07039

CONTENTS

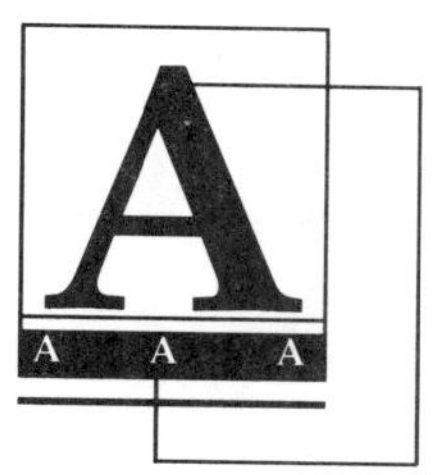

Abortion

Abortion may be either spontaneous (occurring from natural causes) or induced. Since 1980, the number of induced legal abortions reported to Centers for Disease Control has remained fairly stable, varying each year by less than 3 percent.

American Life League (A.L.L.) — *1-703-659-4171*
P.O. Box 1350
Stafford, VA 22554

Purpose This is the largest pro-life, pro-family educational organization in the United States. It provides library research as well as speakers on any of the life issues.

Publications

A.L.L. About Issues, a magazine format covering human interest and information.

Communique, published twice a month, it contains the latest news from the life issues, in both medical and political fields.

Resource list available with over 300 titles covering the whole range of issues.

National Abortion Foundation — *1-800-772-9100*
Pro-Choice Abortion Hotline — *Weekdays 9:30 A.M. to 5:30 P.M. EST*
1436 U St., N.W. — *1-800-424-2280*
Washington, D.C. 20009 — *(in Canada only)*

Purpose The Foundation provides facts about abortion, counseling, and referrals to member clinics.

Abuse

The true statistics on abuse of family members is unknown because so many suffer in silence. One major cause of unreasonable anger is an exaggerated feeling of insecurity and threat. In a society with so many broken families, insecure employment, attacks on self-worth, and other frustrations, the tendency to "take it out" on those nearest is all too common. There is help available for not only the abused but the abuser.

FAMILY VIOLENCE AND SEXUAL ASSAULT INSTITUTE (FVSAI) *1-903-595-6600*
1310 Clinic Drive
Tyler, TX 75701

Purpose The Institute was established in 1984 as a national clearinghouse for research concerning spouse abuse and sexual abuse; to network hospitals, crisis centers, shelters, mental health agencies, practitioners, and researchers; and to provide current research and treatment information. The FVSAI currently has computer reference lists of over 2,000 articles and papers on domestic violence, including spouse abuse, child physical abuse, sexual abuse, and elder abuse. In addition, the FVSAI conducts research treatment programs for spouse abuse and sexual abuse, reviews materials, publishes treatment manuals, and provides consulting services to organizations and agencies.

Publications

Brochures that describe the program.

Treatment manuals on spouse abuse prevention and support for battered and formerly battered women.

Family Violence Bulletin, a quarterly newsletter.

NATIONAL COUNCIL ON CHILD ABUSE (NCCA) *1-800-222-2000 Hotline*
1155 Connecticut Ave., N.W., Suite 300
Washington, D.C. 20036

NATIONAL INSTITUTE OF MENTAL HEALTH (NIMH) *1-301-443-2403*
Information Resources and Inquiries Branch *Fax 1-301-443-0008*
Office of Scientific Information, Room 15C
5900 Fishers Lane, Room 15-105
Rockville, MD 20857

Publication

Plain Talk About Wife Abuse, ADM 85-1265, a 3-page pamphlet.

PARENTS ANONYMOUS *1-213-388-6685 Administration*
520 S. Lafayette Park, Room 316 *1-800-421-0353 Parent stressline (24 hours)*
Los Angeles, CA 80057

Purpose To provide parents safe access to information, support, and referrals to Parents Anonymous services and other resources where applicable. There are available Parents Anonymous support groups, child care and children's groups, and programs for the entire family. It does not refer to physicians or therapists in private practice, but it does refer to self-help groups and/or mental health agencies.

Publications
List of booklets, books, and videotapes available for sale.

SURVIVORS OF INCEST ANONYMOUS, INC. (SIA) *1-410-433-2365*
P.O. Box 21817
Baltimore, MD 21222

Purpose The SIA offers a 12-step, self-help recovery program for adult survivors of child sexual abuse. SIA defines incest very broadly. There are no dues or fees. It makes referrals to support groups, offers pen pals for support, and provides speakers.

Publications
Send a stamped, self-addressed envelope for:

Bi-monthly bulletins.

Survivors of Incest Anonymous, a brochure that includes the 12 steps.

Survivors of Incest literature order form.

Survivors of Incest Anonymous: Survivors Reaching Out to Survivors, a brochure.

ACUPUNCTURE

Chinese medicine maintains there is a pattern of energy called *chi* that is essential to well-being. This energy is believed to flow through the body in meridians, or channels, each day. The acupuncturists deal with 14 of these meridians and up to 1,000 points along them. The acupuncturist inserts thin needles at certain points, usually to interrupt pain. The therapy is said to work by adjusting the energy flow along the meridians.

INTERNATIONAL COLLEGE OF ACUPUNCTURE AND ELECTRO-THERAPEUTICS *1-212-781-6262*
Weekdays 10 A.M. to 10 P.M. EST
800 Riverside Drive, Apt. 8-I
New York, NY 10032

Purpose This nonprofit education organization chartered by the University of the State of New York provides acupuncture and electrotherapy training courses for physicians, dentists, and related health professionals, accredited toward requirements for practicing acupuncture by the New York State Boards for Medicine and Dentistry. During the teaching and training sessions, elected patients are diagnosed and treated for free by volunteer faculty. The College promotes research and teaching of safe and effective acupuncture and electrotherapeutics and related treatments, including Qi Gong and herbal medicine. It aims to combine the best of Western and Oriental medicine through international cooperation and inform the medical profession and the public about the potential benefits as well as adverse effects of these treatments.

ADDISON'S DISEASE

The production of hormones by the outer layer of the adrenal gland lying above the kidneys gradually decreases in this condition. The most common cause of the disease is destruction of the outer layer by the body itself, an autoimmune condition. Tuberculosis, tumors, or inflammation may also cause the disease. Symptoms include

- Weakness and fatigue
- Feeling faint or dizzy when standing up
- Tanning of the skin and other skin discolorations

NATIONAL INSTITUTE OF DIABETES AND DIGESTIVE AND KIDNEY DISEASES (NIDDKD) — *1-301-499-3583*
Building 31, Room 9A04
Bethesda, MD 20892

Publication
Addison's Disease, NIH Pub. No. 90-3054.

ADOPTION

See also Infertility *and* Pregnancy.

Loving and raising a child does not mean you have to be the biological parent. Adoption is an alternative for many infertile couples. The number of children available for adoption has decreased dramatically over the past two decades. The waiting list for Caucasian babies may be as long as seven years. The majority of adoptions today take place through social agencies, but there are still many "private adoptions."

GLADNEY CENTER — *1-800-GLADNEY*
Maternity Home and Infant Placement Center — *Maternity inquiries hotline*
2300 Hemphill — *1-817-922-6000 Adoption inquiries*
Fort Worth, TX 76110

Purpose The Center offers residential or nonresidential maternity programs for young women facing unplanned pregnancy and considering the adoption option. It also provides adoption services to infertile couples and postadoption services to all members of the adoption triad. Gladney will provide housing, if needed, as well as medical care, counseling, education, career development, and legal and postadoption services, all at no charge to birth mother who makes an adoption plan. The Center will make referrals to physicians and self-help groups.

Publications

An American Crisis, a video for medical and counseling professionals with overview of teen pregnancy crisis in America and presentation of options to the crisis pregnancy.

Discover Gladney, a brochure that describes various aspects of program for birth and adoptive mothers.

Presenting Options for Crisis Pregnancy.

AEROBICS

See Physical Fitness.

AGING

See also Alcoholism and Elderly.

There are more Americans over 65 years than under 25 years for the first time in history, and the average age is steadily increasing. People over 65 now represent about 12 percent of the U.S. population and utilize about 30 percent of all health care resources; these figures are projected to reach over 20 percent and 50 percent, respectively, by 2030.

AGING NETWORK SERVICES *1-301-986-1608*
4400 East West Highway, Suite 907
Bethesda, MD 20014

Purpose The Services provide referral to agencies that will meet your needs in your state.

CHILDREN OF AGING PARENTS (CAPS) *1-215-945-6900*
Woodbourne Office Campus, Suite 302-A
1609 Woodbourne Rd.
Levittown, PA 19057

Purpose CAPS provides resource information on long-distance caregiving, family caregiving issues and concerns, respite care, informal support systems, housing and care facilities, understanding the elderly, social services, legal issues and referral services, long-term care issues, and adult day care services.

Publications

CAPS flyer.

CAPS Publication Lists f Caregiving Issues and Concerns.

The Capsule, a bimonthly newsletter available through membership.

Caregiving, information sheet on some problems that affect caregivers.

Care Sharing Directory.

What Does CAPS Do? an information sheet.

COUNCIL ON FAMILY HEALTH — *1-212-598-3617*
225 Park Avenue South, Suite 1700
New York, NY 10003

Publication

Medicines and You: A Guide for Older Americans.

FAMILY CAREGIVER
P.O. Box 15329
Stamford, CT 06901

Publication

Send a large, self-addressed, stamped envelope for

The Family Caregiver, a brochure by Carol A. Miller, M.S.N., R.N.C., an expert working with older adults and their families, developed under a grant from Vicks Vapor Rub. Contains a medication use chart.

LIGHTHOUSE NATIONAL CENTER FOR VISION AND AGING
800 2nd Ave.
New York, NY 10017

1-212-808-0077
1-800-334-5497
Weekdays 9 A.M. to 5 P.M.
(answering machine at other times)
1-808-5544 TDD

Purpose The Lighthouse serves as a national clearinghouse for information on vision and aging. It provides information to consumers and professionals about specific eye disorders and/or professional materials. The Lighthouse also provides consumer resources for large print books, recorded reading materials, and electronic magnification/computer devices. The Center refers consumers to low-vision centers, rehabilitation agencies, and support groups within their locale. It also provides information and/or referral and publications for older people with hearing loss.

Publications

Single copies of the following may be obtained at no cost:

Aging and Vision News, a newsletter published three times a year by the Lighthouse National Center for Vision and Aging, offers interesting articles related to vision and aging for professionals engaged in research, education, and service delivery.

A Better View of You, a brochure in English and Spanish that contains information for older people about age-related eye diseases and low vision.

Lighthouse Low-Vision Products Catalog, a loose-leaf binder that contains descriptions of a wide range of optical devices, products, and services for the low-vision practitioner.

Lighthouse National Center for Vision and Aging, a brochure that describes the mission and activities of the National Center for Vision and Aging.

Low-Vision Continuing Education, a catalog that describes courses in all aspects of low-vision care available for ophthalmologists, optometrists, opticians, registered nurses, technicians, administrators; externship for optometry students; course for ophthalmology residents; and a consultation program to help analyze low-vision practice potential.

Low-Vision Information, a photographic essay on partial-sight picture scenes and text as viewed by persons with cataract, corneal disease, macular degeneration, diabetic retinopathy, glaucoma, retinitis pigmentosa, and hemianopia.

Sound & Sight, a brochure in English or Spanish that provides information about age-related hearing and vision loss.

Work Sight, one brochure for employers-managers, another for employees. These brochures focus on age-related vision disability and how visually impaired older workers can remain in the workplace. Useful for employee health promotion and wellness programs and for vision rehabilitation agencies working with employers.

NATIONAL ACADEMY OF ELDER LAW ATTORNEYS
655 N. Alvernon, Room 108
Tucson, AZ 85711

Publication

Send a stamped, self-addressed envelope to the Academy for *Questions and Answers When Looking for an Elder Law Attorney,* a free brochure.

NATIONAL COUNCIL ON AGING (NCOA) — *1-202-479-1200*
409 Third St., S.W., 2nd floor — *Fax 1-202-479-0735*
Washington, D.C. 20024

Purpose Established in 1950, the NCOA is a private, nonprofit organization with a membership of individual, voluntary agencies, associations, business organizations, labor unions, and others united by a common commitment to improve the lives of older Americans. NCOA forms cooperative relations with government, business, private foundations, and other funding sources to demonstrate the validity of new ideas and services to educate the public and professionals about them and to anticipate and signal challenges and opportunities of the future. Field offices in New York City and Los Angeles offer assignments, training, and placement of older workers.

Publications

Abstracts in Social Gerontology: Current Literature on Aging, a free quarterly annotated bibliography that presents the most recent books, articles, and periodicals on gerontology.

Perspectives on Aging, a free award-winning bimonthly magazine.

NATIONAL INSTITUTE ON AGING (NIA)

Public Inquiries
Federal Building, Room 6C12
Bethesda, MD 20892

The National Institute on Aging is charged with the responsibility for the conduct and support of biomedical, social, and behavioral research and training related to the aging process and the diseases and other special problems and needs of the aged. The NIA supports research on osteoporosis and related topics, such as bone loss, falls, and hip fractures, which are major causes of frailty and dependence experienced among the older population.

Publications

Free copies of the following "Age Pages" are available.

Accidents and the Elderly. (Also available in Spanish.)
Aging and Alcohol Abuse.
Aging and Your Eyes.
AIDS and Older Adults.
Arthritis Advice. (Also available in Chinese.)
Be Sensible About Salt.
Can Life Be Extended?
Cancer Facts for People over 50. (Also available in Chinese.)
Considering Surgery?
Constipation. (Also available in Chinese.)
Crime and the Elderly. (Also available in Spanish.)
Dealing with Diabetes. (Also available in Chinese and Spanish.)
Dietary Supplements: More Is Not Always Better. (Also available in Chinese.)
Digestive Do's and Don'ts. (Also available in Spanish.)
Don't Take It Easy—Exercise!
Finding Good Medical Care.
Foot Care for Older People. (Also available in Chinese and Spanish.)
Getting Your Affairs in Order.
Health Quackery.
Heat, Cold, and Being Old. (Also available in Spanish.)

High Blood Pressure: A Common but Controllable Disorder. (Also available in Chinese.)
Hints for Shopping, Cooking, and Enjoying Meals.
A Hot Weather Hazard for Older People: Hyperthermia, NIH Pub. No. 89-2763.
The National Institute on Aging, NIH Pub. No. 83-1129.
Nutrition: A Lifelong Concern. (Also available in Chinese and Spanish.)
Osteoporosis: The Bone Thinner.
Preventing Falls and Fractures.
Prostate Problems.
Q&A Alzheimer's Disease, NIH Pub. No. 80-1646.
Safe Use of Medicines by Older People. (Also available in Chinese.)
Safe Use of Tranquilizers.
Safety Belt Sense.
Senility: Myth or Madness?
Sexuality in Later Life.
Should You Take Estrogen?
Skin Care and Aging. (Also available in Spanish.)
Smoking: It's Never Too Late to Stop.
Taking Care of Your Teeth and Mouth.
Urinary Incontinence.
What Is Your Aging IQ?
What to Do About the Flu. (Also available in Chinese.)
When You Need a Nursing Home.
Who's Who in Health Care. (Also available in Spanish.)
A Winter Hazard for Older People: Accidental Hypothermia, NIH Pub. No. 86-1464.

NATIONAL INSTITUTES OF HEALTH (NIH) *1-301-496-2563*
Office of Clinical Center Communications
Building 10, Room 1C255
Bethesda, MD 20892

Publication

Coping with Aging Parents, (a videotape that can be borrowed).

AIDS (AUTOIMMUNE DEFICIENCY SYNDROME)

See also National Gay and Lesbian Task Force *under* Sexually Transmitted Diseases.

AIDS (acquired immunodeficiency syndrome) is caused by the human immunodeficiency virus (HIV) and leads to a weakening of the immune system, which in turn results in opportunistic infections, malignancies, and neurological lesions.

Desert Stream Ministries *1-213-572-0140*
AIDS Resource Ministry
12488 Venice Blvd.
Los Angeles, CA 90066-3804

Purpose This organization has support groups for persons with HIV; a group for family and friends; visitation ministry for persons with HIV and equipping church to minister to persons impacted by HIV.

Publications
General information about the ministry.

Homosexual Information Center *1-318-742-4709*
115 Monroe
Bossier City, LA 71111-4539

Purpose The Center provides information about HIV/AIDS.

Publication
Notes on AIDS.

J2CP Information Services
P.O. Box 184
San Juan Capistrano, CA 92693-0184

Bulletin Board System

Line 1: 1-714-248-2836
U.S. Robotics HST Dual Standard
9600/2400/1200/300, 8N1
Full Duplex

Line 2: 1-714-248-2866
U.S. Robotics HST Dual Standard
9600/2400/1200/300 8N1
Full Duplex

Purpose The Sisters of St. Elizabeth operate J2CP Information Services and the HIV/AIDS information bulletin board system. J2CP's outreach includes information and referrals. However, its data library and referral information are available only through computer bulletin boards. Information available addresses legal, medical, political, psychological, and religious issues related to transsexualism. A state-by-state referral list will also be available. Additionally, the subboard (type B to access from the main menu) will be tied into the international Gender Dysphoria echo-mail conference. The HIV/AIDS information bulletin board, in addition to providing a link to the international AIDS/ARC echo-mail conference, provides an extensive data library on HIV/AIDS and support services referral director. Access is free. The bulletin board is capable of receiving calls from anywhere in the world.

National AIDS Hotline

1-800-342-AIDS 7 days a week, 24 hours a day
1-800-344-SIDA Spanish 7 days a week, 8 A.M.-2 A.M. EST
1-800-AIDS-TTY Hearing impaired, 10 A.M.-10 P.M. EST

Purpose The National AIDS Hotline (NAH) is a toll-free service available to the general public 24 hours a day, 7 days a week throughout the United States and its territories. Operated since 1986 by the American Social Health Association (ASHA), under contract with the National AIDS Information and Education Program of the Centers for Disease Control (CDC), the hotline provides callers with confidential information and referrals related to AIDS and HIV infection. Trained information specialists are available to answer calls in English and Spanish or through a TTY/TDD machine for the deaf and hard-of-hearing. The specialists can answer questions about HIV transmission, AIDS prevention, risk reduction behaviors (including abstinence, safer sex, and needle usage), HIV antibody testing, symptoms, treatment, resources, and other topics. Callers can be given referrals specific to their needs, including public health clinics and hospitals, alternative HIV-test site locations, counseling and support groups, AIDS educational organizations, local hotlines, financial and legal services, and many others. Hotline staff also arrange for mailing of free CDC-approved printed materials, including pamphlets and posters. Certain services are available to the deaf by staff capable of communicating in American and English Sign Languages (ASL and ESL). Certain services are also available in Spanish. Financial referrals to individuals; legal referrals.

National Center for Research Resources

1-301-496-5545

Westwood Building, Room 857
Bethesda, MD 20892

Publication
AIDS in Children.

National Institute of Allergy and Infectious Diseases (NIAID)

1-800-TRIALS-A
Weekdays 9 A.M. to 5 P.M. EST

The AIDS Clinical Trials Information Service
Building 31, Room 7A32
Bethesda, MD 20892

Purpose The NIAID provides information about AIDS/HIV clinical trials conducted by the National Institutes of Health and other FDA-approved trials.

Publication
AIDS Clinical Trials: Talking It Over, NIH Pub. No. 89-3025. Also available in Spanish (NIH Pub. No. 89-3025).

NATIONAL INSTITUTE OF MENTAL HEALTH (NIMH) *1-301-443-2403*
Information Resources and Inquiries Branch *Fax 1-301-443-0008*
Office of Scientific Information, Room 15C
5900 Fishers Lane, Room 15-105
Rockville, MD 20857

Publication
When Someone Close Has AIDS: Acquired Immunodeficiency Syndrome, ADM 89 1515, 15 pages.

NATIONAL INSTITUTES OF HEALTH (NIH) *1-301-496-2563*
Office of Clinical Center Communications
Building 10, Room 1C255
Bethesda, MD 20892

Publication
AIDS: Can I Catch It?

NEW JERSEY AIDS HOTLINE *1-201-926-7443*
201 Lyons Avenue *1-800-624-2377*
Newark, NJ 07112

Purpose This hotline provides information regarding AIDS—infection, treatment, and testing. Telephone advice and referral for treatment and testing.

Publications
A wide variety.

ALCOHOLISM

An alcoholic is dependent on or addicted to alcohol. The following are symptoms of a serious drinking problem:

- Frequent intoxication
- Waking up in the morning and not remembering what happened the night before
- Blackouts
- Marriage failure
- Work absenteeism and job loss
- Driving while intoxicated
- Physical injuries
- Disorders such as cirrhosis of the liver and delirium tremens

ADULT CHILDREN OF ALCOHOLICS (ACOA) INTERIM WORLD SERVICE ORGANIZATION *1-310-534-1815*
2522 W. Sepulveda Blvd., Suite 200
P.O. Box 3216
Torrance, CA 90505

Purpose Adult Children of Alcoholics is a fellowship of men and women with the common bond of having to recover from the effects of alcoholism. ACOA draws on the Alcoholics Anonymous and Al-Anon family groups' recovery approach. The goal is to make possible emotional sobriety and spiritual freedom for anyone affected by family alcoholism.

AL-ANON FAMILY GROUPS HEADQUARTERS, INC. *1-212-302-7240*
P.O. Box 862, Midtown Station *Fax 1-212-869-3757*
New York, NY 10018-0862 *1-800-356-9996*
24-hour toll-free

Purpose Al-Anon is a 12-step, self-help program for families and friends who have been affected by someone else's drinking. Members share their experience, strength, and hope with each other to help solve their common problems. Al-Anon and Alateen (for younger members) are self-supporting; contributions are voluntary. Al-Anon has no opinions on outside issues and no affiliations and makes no referrals except to its affiliates in other locales.

Publications

Literature and a listing of Al-Anon information services and a catalog listing publications for which there is a charge.

ALATEEN *1-212-302-7240*
P.O. Box 862, Midtown Station *Fax 1-212-869-3757*
New York, NY 10018-0862 *1-800-356-9996*
24-hour toll-free

Purpose For those 15 to 20 years old who live in an alcoholic family situation to learn effective ways to cope with problems, aims, for loving detachment from alcoholic family.

ALCOHOL, DRUG ABUSE, AND MENTAL HEALTH ADMINISTRATION *1-301-443-4795*
Parklawn Building
5600 Fishers Lane
Rockville, MD 20857

ALCOHOL REHAB FOR THE ELDERLY
P.O. Box 267
Hopedale, IL 61747

1-800-354-7089 Hotline
1-800-344-0824 (Illinois only)

ALCOHOLICS ANONYMOUS (AA)
475 Riverside Drive, 11th floor
New York, NY 10115

1-212-870-3400
Fax 1-212-870-3003

Purpose Alcoholics Anonymous is a voluntary worldwide fellowship of men and women who meet to attain and maintain sobriety through its 12-step program of recovery and "12 Traditions." AA's primary purpose is to help alcoholics stay sober and achieve sobriety.

ALCOHOLISM AND DRUG ADDICTION
TREATMENT CENTER
McDonald Center/Scripps Memorial Hospital
9904 Genesee Ave.
La Jolla, CA 92037

1-800-382-4357

FAMILIES ANONYMOUS (FA)
P.O. Box 528
Van Nuys, CA 91408

1-800-736-9805

Purpose Founded in 1971, by a group of Los Angeles families, FA bases its approach on the 12 steps of Alcoholics Anonymous. This self-help group consists of families of drug or alcohol abusers and those with behavioral problems. The focus of the program is on the family in crisis, not the user. It is not drug or behavior specific. Many newcomers arrive in crisis with a child, spouse, or friend in jail or a recovery or rehab facility. The goal is to allow families to put their lives together and find a sense of serenity. FA focuses on the member's recovery or change in attitudes and reactions. Emotions such as anger, fear, guilt, and resentment, FA believes, retard recovery. It will refer to other self-help groups when appropriate, but these must be "12 step."

Publications
Booklets, bookmarks, posters, and audio tape formats.

NATIONAL CLEARINGHOUSE FOR ALCOHOL AND
DRUG INFORMATION (NCADI)
P.O. Box 2345
Rockville, MD 20852

1-301-468-2600

Publications

The National Clearinghouse for Alcohol and Drug Information: A New National Resource, MS219, describes NCADI services.

Taking Care of Your Baby Before Birth, PH239A, targeted to low-income pregnant women, this pamphlet describes alcohol's effects on the baby, alternatives to drinking, and sources for help.

What You Can Do About Drug Use in America, PHD507A, an introductory brochure that calls individuals to action and to making a commitment to participate in creating protective, drug-free communities for youth.

Drug-Free Communities: Turning Awareness into Action, PHD519A, helps parents and other adult groups come to a shared understanding of alcohol and other drug problems as a concern that affects the entire community.

NATIONAL COUNCIL ON ALCOHOLISM AND DRUG DEPENDENCE (NCADD)
Attn: Information Director
12 W. 21st St.
New York, NY 10010

1-212-206-6770
Fax 1-212-645-1690
1-800-NCA-CALL

Purpose The National Council on Alcoholism and Drug Dependence, Inc., is a national nonprofit organization combating alcoholism, other drug addictions, and related problems. Founded in 1944, NCADD's major programs include prevention and education, public information, medical/scientific information, public policy, advocacy, and publications. NCADD's network of nearly 200 affiliates conducts similar activities at the state and local levels and provides information and referral services to families and individuals seeking help with an alcohol or other drug problem. When the toll-free telephone number is called, the caller is given the telephone number of the nearest NCADD affiliate or other referral resource and mailed general information about alcoholism or teen-specified information.

SEVENTH-DAY ADVENTIST COMMUNITY HEALTH SERVICES
P.O. Box 1029
Manhasset, NY 11030

1-516-627-2210

Publication

The Mocker, facing alcoholism with the 12 steps endorsed biblically.

SOS/SECULAR ORGANIZATION FOR SOBRIETY/ SAVE OUR SELVES
P.O. Box 5
Buffalo, NY 14215-0005

1-716-834-2922
24-hour phone

Purpose SOS is an alternative recovery method for those alcoholics or drug addicts who are uncomfortable with the spiritual content of widely available 12-step programs. SOS takes a reasonable, secular approach to recovery and maintains that sobriety is a separate issue from religion or spirituality. SOS credits the individual for achieving and maintaining his or her own sobriety. SOS respects recovery in any form, regardless of the path by which it is achieved. It is a network of nonprofit, autonomous, nonprofessional local groups dedicated solely to helping individuals achieve and maintain sobriety. Will refer to self-help groups and physicians.

Publications
Secular Organizations for Sobriety, a brochure.
Save Ourselves: Recovery for Families and Friends of Alcoholics and Addicts, a brochure.
Save Ourselves: The Sobriety Priority, a brochure.
Save Ourselves: Your First Thirty Days, a brochure.
SOS National Newsletter.

ALLERGY

The word *allergy* is a comparatively new one, since it has been used for little more than 75 years. It is derived from the Greek word *allos*, meaning "altered," and *ergia*, meaning "reactivity." The conditions that cause an allergic response, however, are as old as humankind. Hieroglyphics describe the death of King Menes of Egypt in 2641 B.C. from the sting of a wasp. There are 35 million allergy sufferers in the United States, according to the National Institutes of Health, and many are not aware that there are new methods of preventing, diagnosing, and treating allergies. They do not know that they no longer need suffer with an itchy rash or a chronically stuffed nose. They do not have to fight to get air into their lungs. Recent advances in science have revealed new information about how the body musters its defenses against invaders and have led to improvements in diagnosis and therapy of allergies.

ALLERGY INFORMATION CENTER AND HOTLINE *1-800-727-5400*

Purpose Sponsored by Fisons Corporation, makers of Nasalcrom®, a prescription remedy for allergic rhinitis, the company offers free booklets and referrals to physicians' association and allergy support groups nationwide.

Publications
Allergy Calendar.
Allergy Sufferer's Guide to the Great Outdoors.
Are Allergies in Your Family Tree?
Consumer's Guide to Allergy Medications.
A Consumer's Guide to Indoor Allergies.
Do You Know Your Allergy Potential?
U.S. Pollen Predictor.
Welcome to the Allergy Neighborhood Coloring Book.

AMERICAN ACADEMY OF ALLERGY AND IMMUNOLOGY
611 East Wells Street
Milwaukee, WI 53202

1-414-272-6071
1-800-822-ASMA Hotline

Purpose The American Academy of Allergy and Immunology advances the knowledge and practice of allergy, fosters the education of students and the public, encourages union and cooperation among those working in the field, and promotes and stimulates research and the study of allergic disease. Referrals are made to physicians in your area or to self-help groups. Responds to requests for information.

Publications

Childhood Asthma. See also Asthma.

The Asthma & Allergy Advocate, a quarterly newsletter for the allergy sufferer. *See also* Asthma.

Tips to Remember Series, colorful pamphlets containing educational information on asthma and allergies for the lay audience.

AMERICAN ACADEMY OF OTOLARYNGOLOGY HEAD AND NECK SURGERY (AAOHNS)
One Prince Street
Alexandria, VA 22314

1-703-836-4444
Fax 703-683-5100

Publications

Send a stamped, self-addressed envelope for

Hayfever, Summer Colds and Allergies.

You and Your Stuffy Nose.

See American Academy of Dermatology listed *under* Skin, for brochures on allergic contact rashes and eczema.

AMERICAN ACADEMY OF PEDIATRICS
P.O. Box 927
Elk Grove Village, IL 60009-0927

Publication

Send a self-addressed, stamped, business-size envelope to Department C for

Allergies in Children: Plain Talk for Parents.

CONSUMER GUIDE TO TREATING ALLERGIES
P.O. Box 731
Radio City Station
New York, NY 10101-0731

Publication

Send a self-addressed stamped envelope for

Consumer Guide to Treating Allergies, a 14-page booklet containing "must avoid" side effects of medication and definitions.

FOOD ALLERGY CENTER *1-800-YES-RELIEF*
53-31 Marathon Parkway
Little Neck, NY 11362

Purpose The Center is a resource for people in need of general information pertaining to food allergies and sensitivities. Callers receive information on food allergies, including alternatives for testing and treatments. No diagnosis can be made. Referrals are made to physicians and self-help groups.

Publications

FAN, food allergy newsletter. Helpful information and tips for the food allergic, including recipes. First issue free.

The Food Allergy Center Brochure: A Guide to Food Allergies and Their Treatment.

NATIONAL ALLERGY AND ASTHMA NETWORK/ *1-703-385-4403*
MOTHERS OF ASTHMATICS, INC. *1-800-878-4403 Hotline*
3554 Chain Bridge Rd., Suite 200
Fairfax, VA 22030

Purpose This organization is a nonprofit health association dedicated to assisting millions of patients with asthma and allergies. It provides support and guidance with a toll-free hotline.

Publications

List of asthma and allergy resources.

The MA Newsletter, a monthly.

NATIONAL FOUNDATION FOR THE *1-517-697-3989*
CHEMICALLY HYPERSENSITIVE
P.O. Box 9
Wrightsville Beach, NC 28480-0009

Purpose The Foundation is a nonprofit, volunteer organization devoted to research, education, and dissemination of information about chemical hypersensitivity. Referrals are made to physicians and attorneys. Advice and resource assistance for the chemically injured and their relatives are provided.

Publication
Brochure on the National Foundation for the Chemically Hypersensitive.

NATIONAL INSTITUTE OF ALLERGY AND INFECTIOUS DISEASES (NIAID) *1-301-496-5717*
Building 31, Room 7A32
Bethesda, MD 20892

Publications
Asthma, NIH Pub. No. 83-525. See also Asthma.
Drug Allergy, NIH Pub. No. 82-703.
Dust Allergy, NIH Pub. No. 83-490.
Mold Allergy, NIH Pub. No. 84-797.
NAID: The Edge of Discovery, NIH Pub. No. 8802773.
Poison Ivy Allergy, NIH Pub. No. 82-897.
Pollen Allergy, NIH Pub. No. 87-493.

NATIONAL INSTITUTES OF HEALTH *1-301-496-2563*
Office Of Clinical Center Communications
Building 10, Room 1C255
Bethesda, MD 20892

Publications
Allergic Diseases, Pub. No. 91-3221.
Allergic Diseases, (a videotape that can be borrowed free of charge).

NATIONAL JEWISH CENTER FOR IMMUNOLOGY AND RESPIRATORY MEDICINE *1-800-222-5864*
1400 Jackson Street
Denver, CO 80206

Purpose This agency is a specialty medical center dedicated to the treatment of respiratory, allergic, and immunologic disorders.

Publications
Air pollution and Asthma.
Allergies.
Asthma. (See also Asthma.)
Chronic Bronchitis.
Chronic Cough.
Emphysema.

Interstitial Lung Disease.
Juvenile Rheumatoid Arthritis.
Lupus.
Mycobacterial Diseases.
Occupational Lung Diseases.
Pneumonia.
Sleep Disorders.
Smoking.
Steroids—Side Effects.
Tuberculosis.
Vocal Cord Dysfunction.

SCHERING-PLOUGH INC.
P.O. Box 5129
Dept. MAT
Bergenfield, NJ 07621

Publication
The Official Chlor-Trimeton Handbook for the Allergic Athlete.

ALZHEIMER'S

Alzheimer's is a progressive degenerative disease that attacks the brain and results in impaired memory, thinking, and behavior. It affects an estimated 2.5 million American adults. Alzheimer's usually has a gradual onset. Problems remembering recent events and difficulty performing familiar tasks are early symptoms. Additionally, the Alzheimer patient also may experience confusion, personality change, behavior change, impaired judgment, and difficulty finding words, finishing thoughts, or following directions. How quickly these changes occur will vary from person to person, but the disease eventually leaves its victims totally unable to care for themselves. Not all persons experiencing the symptoms just listed have Alzheimer's and may have an easily treatable condition. Therefore, proper diagnosis is imperative, requiring medical, neurologic, and psychiatric evaluations, as well as neuropsychological tests.

ALZHEIMER'S ASSOCIATION *1-312-335-8700*
919 North Michigan Avenue, Suite 1000 *1-800-272-3900*
Chicago, IL 60611-1676 *1-312-335-8882 TDD*
Fax 1-312-335-1110

Purpose This national nonprofit organization is dedicated to research for the prevention, cure, and treatment of Alzheimer's disease and related disorders and to provide support and assistance to afflicted patients and their families. The goals of the Association include research into the cause, prevention, treatment, and cure for

Alzheimer's disease and related disorders; education of the public and information for health care professionals; formation for a nationwide family support network and implementation of programs at the local level; and advocacy for improved public policy and needed legislation and patient and family service to aid present and future victims and caregivers. The Association operates a toll-free information and referral service to send free literature to callers requesting information on Alzheimer's disease and related disorders. Callers will also be given the phone number of the local chapter in their area, where they can receive information about support groups and the patient and family services available to them.

Publications

The Alzheimer's Disease Newsletter, distributed quarterly.
A number of other publications on the subject are available, (some in Spanish).

NATIONAL INSTITUTE OF HEALTH (NIH) *1-301-496-2563*
Office of Clinical Center Communications
Building 10, Room 1C255
Bethesda, MD 20892

Publication

Alzheimer's Disease, NIH Pub. No. 88-2982.

For further information on Alzheimer's disease and related disorders, write to:

National Institute on Aging (NIA)
Alzheimer's Disease Education and Referral (ADEAR) Center
NIAC, P.O. Box 8250
Silver Spring, MD 20907

NATIONAL INSTITUTE OF MENTAL HEALTH (NIMH) *1-301-443-2403*
Information Resources and Inquiries Branch *Fax 1-301-443-0008*
Office of Scientific Information, Room 15C
5900 Fishers Lane, Room 15-105
Rockville, MD 20857

Publications

There Were Times, Dear . . . Living with Alzheimer's Disease, OM 87-4023, 21 pages.

Useful Information on Alzheimer's Disease, ADM 90-1696, 24 pages.

AMYOTROPHIC LATERAL SCLEROSIS (ALS)

A disease of unknown cause, it involves muscular weakness and atrophy. It usually occurs after age 40 and more frequently in men than women.

AMYOTROPHIC LATERAL SCLEROSIS ASSOCIATION (ALSA) *1-818-340-7500*
21021 Ventura Blvd. *1-800-782-4747 Hotline*
Woodland Hills, CA 91364

Purpose The Association is a nonprofit, tax-exempt, voluntary national health organization dedicated solely to finding the cause, treatment, and cure of amyotrophic lateral sclerosis (Lou Gehrig's disease). ALS helps people with the condition and their families through referrals for counseling, training, and support on how to cope with this devastating disease, providing clinical care regardless of race, color, creed, or financial status through its nationwide network of ALSA Centers. It serves as the national information center on ALS for medical professionals, patients, and family members.

Publications

LINK, a quarterly newsletter.

MALS Manual I—Finding Help, a realistic introduction for patients and family members coping with ALS. Stresses the importance of reliable, current information about the disease. Includes recommendations of available agencies and health care services that provide guidance and/or assistance.

MALS Manual II—Managing Muscle Weakness, keys in on the difficulties in walking and full muscle use of ALS patients. Includes information on exercise, assistance devices, canes and walkers, wheelchairs and lifters, and recovery from falls.

MALS Manual III—Managing Breathing Problems, covers the importance of preventative measures needed to maintain optimal lung capacity. Discusses direct breathing aids when breathing muscles weaken.

MALS Manual IV—Managing Swallowing Problems, suggests types of food and proper body alignment to help alleviate swallowing difficulties. Discusses alternative methods of eating and nutrition as swallowing difficulties progress.

MALS Manual V—Managing Communication Problems, discusses ways for ALS patients to prolong speaking ability through such methods as slower articulation and palate lift. Augmentative communication techniques are detailed, including eye movement, communication boards, and special computer programs.

Michael Gross Speaks about ALS.

What is Amyotrophic Lateral Sclerosis?

NATIONAL INSTITUTE OF NEUROLOGICAL *1-301-496-5751*
DISORDERS AND STROKE (NINDS)
Building 31, Room 8A06
Bethesda, MD 20892

Publication

Amyotrophic Lateral Sclerosis, NIH Pub. No. 84-916.

ANESTHESIA

Anesthesia works by blocking pain. There are three basic types:

- General, in which you are unconscious
- Regional or conduction, including spinal and epidural, in which you are awake but numb in a specific region
- Local, in which you are awake and only the area being operated on is numb

General anesthesia makes you unaware of pain by working on the part of the brain that receives pain signals. Conduction and local anesthesia block the signals sent to the spinal cord and brain from the site which is anesthetized.

Some of the newer anesthetics are combinations of two of the three types listed.

AMERICAN SOCIETY OF ANESTHESIOLOGISTS *1-708-825-5586*
515 Busse Highway
Park Ridge, IL 60068-3189

Purpose The American Society of Anesthesiologists was founded in 1905. It is a scientific and educational association of anesthesiologists that was organized to advance the practice of anesthesiology and to improve the quality of care of the anesthetized patient. It is the largest organization of anesthesiologists in the world with approximately 30,000 members. It does not refer to physicians or self-help groups.

Publications

Single copies of the following are available without charge:

Anesthesia & You, an 8-page newsletter informing what anesthesia is, why it is needed, and the anesthesiologist's role in patient care.

Know Your Anesthesiologist, an 8-page brochure describes what you need to know about good anesthesia care.

The Management of Pain, a brochure that covers topics such as chronic versus acute pain, various medication, therapies, and procedures and explains the role of anesthesiologists in pain management.

The Older Patient, with new advancements in anesthetic agents and monitoring equipment, anesthesiologists have a better understanding of medical problems associated with the aging process. Describes how anesthesiologists apply this knowledge to safely administer anesthesia to the older patient.

Planning Your Childbirth, a 10-page brochure discusses modern anesthesiology choices for a more comfortable childbirth and answers many of the questions expectant mothers may have concerning pain relief during labor and delivery.

My Trip to the Hospital, a 28-page coloring book, designed to make a child feel at ease about going to the hospital. Discusses the child's journey from entering the hospital or ambulatory surgical center, to the administration of anesthesia, recovery, and going home.

ANOREXIA

See Eating Disorders.

ANXIETY

Anxiety is generally thought of as a feeling, a fear of impending danger or damage that makes the heart beat faster, wets the hands with sweat, and even stimulates the involuntary muscles of the intestine and bladder. On one hand, anxiety may be a normal physiological response, an alerting mechanism that prepares the body for action and actually enhances functioning. At the same time, excessive anxiety or anxiety that is misdirected can become a problem that threatens an individual's physical health and impairs or severely disrupts daily functioning. Anxiety is usually considered a disorder when it threatens one's health or interferes with one's functioning at work or at home.

ANXIETY DISORDERS ASSOCIATION OF AMERICA — *1-301-231-9350*
6000 Executive Blvd., Suite 513 — *Fax 1-301-231-7392*
Rockville, MD 20852

Purpose The Anxiety Disorders Association of America, formerly the Phobia Society of America, a nonprofit organization, was founded in 1981. The association is dedicated to educating the public and professionals about the nature of phobias and related anxiety disorders and their treatment, as well as assisting people in locating phobia treatment in their area. The association serves as a national clearinghouse for information on resources and referrals and helps in the exchange of information and ideas on phobia and related anxiety disorders treatment. The organization answers inquiries, provides referrals to psychiatrists, psychologists, other therapists, and self-help Groups.

Publications

ADAA Reporter, newsletter available to members.

NETWORK NEWS, self-help newsletter available to members.

Charges a fee for its many booklets and brochures.

APHASIA

See also Speech

Aphasia is characterized by a defect in or a loss of language function in which the comprehension or expression of words is impaired as a result of injury to the language areas of the brain.

NATIONAL APHASIA ASSOCIATION *1-800-922-4NAA*
P.O. Box 1887
Murray Hill Station
New York, NY 10156-0611

Purpose The Association promotes public awareness of aphasia; improves society's attitudes toward persons with aphasia; increases contact among those with aphasia and among their families; provides information and publications to individuals with aphasia, their families, and interested professionals; stimulates programs that might increase access and availability of support services for persons with aphasia; and promotes research that addresses the improvement of the quality of life for those who have acquired aphasia. It disseminates information about aphasia and refers to local aphasia community groups.

Publications
Send a large, stamped, self-addressed envelope and a donation, if possible, to defray costs for
Aphasia Community Group Manual.
Aphasia Community Groups List.
Aphasia Quiz.
Fact Sheet.
How to Communicate with a Person Who Has Aphasia.
Impact of Aphasia on Patients and Family: Results of a Needs Survey.
Let's Talk.
National Aphasia Association Newsletter, most recent issue complimentary with membership.
National Aphasia Association Question and Answer Sheet.
Press Release/Public Service Announcements.
Regional Representatives.
Selected Readings, a bibliography.
Special Report #1.

NATIONAL INSTITUTE OF NEUROLOGICAL DISORDERS AND STROKE (NINDS) *1-301-496-5751*
Building 31, ROOM 8A06
Bethesda, MD 20892

Publications
Aphasia, NIH Pub. No. 89-391.
Autismo, NIH Pub. No. 81-2282.

ART HAZARDS

Lead poisoning, cancer, miscarriages, nervous system damage, silicosis, chemical pneumonia, asthma, dermatitis—all of these may be found among artists, craftspeople, theater technicians, museum conservators, teachers, and even children who are using art and craft material without adequate precautions. Most of these art-related injuries and illnesses can be prevented through education about the causes of the problems and following suitable precautions.

CENTER FOR SAFETY IN THE ARTS, INC. *1-212-227-6220*
6 Beekman Street
New York, NY 10038

Purpose The Center—formerly the Center for Occupational Hazards—is a national clearinghouse for research and education on hazards in the visual arts, performing arts, educational facilities, and museums. The Center answers approximately 50 written and telephoned inquiries daily on art hazards. Requests for information come from artists, craftspeople, theater technicians, performing artists, teachers, parents, students, museum conservators, physicians, poison control centers, and government agencies. The Center researches the potential hazards of art materials and processes, writes and distributes publications on art hazards, and makes referrals to physicians with expertise in occupational medicine.

Publications

Is Your Art Hurting You? a sheet that explains the mission of the center and the services offered. It also contains an order form for many publications ranging from 50 cents to $16 on specific materials and hazards.

ARTERIOVENOUS MALFORMATION (AVM)

AVM is an abnormal tangled collection of dilated blood vessels that are malformed vascular structures at birth. The malformation may continue to enlarge and may produce neurologic abnormalities either because its size compresses other structures or because it bleeds.

AVM SUPPORT GROUP *1-415-334-8012*
107 Bella Vista Way
San Francisco, CA 94127

Purpose The AVM Support Group provides support to patients with arteriovenous malformation. Family and friends of AVM patients are also involved and supported. Quarterly meetings are held and networking is done. Referrals are made to physicians and to self-help groups.

Publications

General information brochure.
Reprints of articles.
Brochures on treatment options.

ARTHRITIS

See also Lupus.

OSTEOPOROSIS

This condition affects an estimated 24 million Americans, primarily women. It is a debilitating disorder in which the bones deteriorate due to the excessive loss of bone tissue and there is an increased susceptibility to bone fractures. People may not know they have osteoporosis until their bones become so weak that a sudden strain, bump, fall, or routine activity like bending to lift groceries causes a bone fracture.

RHEUMATOID ARTHRITIS

This is an autoimmune disease, that is, a disease in which environmental and/or genetic factors trigger an uncontrollable and destructive reaction by the immune system, directed against the body's own tissues. Population studies have indicated that approximately 1 percent of the adult population is affected with rheumatoid arthritis. The female-to-male ratio is about 2 to 1, and the peak age of incidence is 35 to 55 in males and 40 to 60 in females. The disease is characterized by periods of activity and remission. The damage inflicted is not continuous and ongoing, although it does not necessarily heal perfectly. Joint pain and early morning stiffness are the major symptoms of the disease, and pain is initially felt on movement, but as the disease progresses pain develops at rest.

ARTHRITIS FOUNDATION *1-800-283-7833*
P.O. Box 19000
Atlanta, GA 30326

Purpose The mission of the Arthritis Foundation is to support research to find the cause for and cure for arthritis and to provide services to improve the quality of life for people with arthritis. The chapters may offer not only information but support groups, referral lists of physicians specializing in arthritis, self-help courses, exercise classes, and forums.

Publications

All items are brochures, unless otherwise noted. Single copies of most titles are available free from your local chapter or by writing to the box number given. The Foundation asks that you order no more than three (3) titles at one time.

DAILY LIVING

- ▲ *Arthritis and Employment*, No. 9070, tips for managing arthritis on the job.
- ▲ *Arthritis and Pregnancy*, No. 9331, how arthritis affects pregnancy, and tips for managing pregnancy and a new baby.
- ▲ *Coping with Pain*, No. 9333, describes pain and ways to control it.

- ▲ *Coping with Stress*, No. 9326, describes stress and ways to reduce it.
- ▲ *The Family*, No. 9334, describes the effects of arthritis on family life and ways to cope.
- ▲ *Living and Loving: Information about Sex*, No. 9190, tips for solving problems when arthritis interferes with sexuality.
- ▲ *Practical Information*, No. 4100, where to find help for physical, financial, medical, and legal problems of arthritis.
- ▲ *Taking Charge*, No. 4221, tips for coping with physical and emotional challenges of arthritis.
- ▲ *Travel Tips*, No. 9071, tips for easier land, sea, and air travel.
- ▲ *When Your Student Has Arthritis*, No. 9560, guide for parents and teachers on special problems of children with arthritis in school.

GENERAL INFORMATION

- ▲ *Arthritis and Farmers*, No. 9327, tips for managing arthritis during daily farm activities.
- ▲ *Arthritis & Vocational Rehabilitation*, No. 2250, describes vocational rehabilitation and how to apply.
- ▲ *Arthritis: Do You Know?* (tear-off sheet), No. 5786, overview of arthritis and services of the Arthritis Foundation.
- ▲ *Basic Facts*, No. 4001, an overview of arthritis, common types, and treatments.
- ▲ *Diet*, No. 4280, answers questions about the role of diet in arthritis.
- ▲ *Guide to Effective Volunteer Lobbying*, No. 4012, how to approach legislators about arthritis-related issues.
- ▲ *Guide to Insurance for People with Arthritis*, No. 9332, health, disability, and life insurance information.
- ▲ *Guide to Social Security Disability Insurance for People with Arthritis*, No. 2230, step-by-step information on obtaining benefits.
- ▲ *Help Your Doctor-Help Yourself*, No. 9325, how to strengthen communication with your doctor.
- ▲ *Research: What's New*, No. 4222, advances in research and how to evaluate media reports on research.
- ▲ *Services of the Arthritis Foundation*, No. 4010, lists services and programs available
- ▲ *Unproven Remedies*, No. 4240, defines unproven remedies and how to identify them.

The Arthritis Foundation is the source of help and hope for Americans who have arthritis. Contact your local chapter to find out what services are available in your area.

MATERIALS IN OTHER LANGUAGES

- ▲ *La Arthritis Infantojuvenil*, No. 4165, describes juvenile arthritis and its treatment, Spanish with illustrations.

MEDICATIONS

These brochures describe how medicines work, describing dosages, and possible side effects.

- ▲ *Aspirin*, No. 4260.
- ▲ *Corticosteroid Medications*, No. 9220.
- ▲ *Cytotoxic Drugs*, No. 9040.
- ▲ *Gold Treatment*, No. 4120.
- ▲ *Guide to Medications*, No. 9059.
- ▲ *Hydroxychloroquine (Plaquenil)*, No. 9200.
- ▲ *Nonsteroidal Anti-inflammatory Drugs*, No. 9041.
- ▲ *Penicillamine (Cuprimine, Depen)*, No. 9300.

TREATMENTS

- ▲ *Exercise and Your Arthritis*, No. 9704, types of exercise for people with arthritis and how to do them.
- ▲ *Guide to Laboratory Tests*, No. 9060, lists common tests to diagnose and monitor arthritis.
- ▲ *Guide to Medications*, No. 9059, general tips about medicines and how to take them safely.
- ▲ *Surgery*, No. 4230, information about joint surgery.
- ▲ *Taking Care: Joint Protection*, No. 9329, tips on methods and devices for protecting joints.

TYPES OF ARTHRITIS

These brochures explain what is currently understood about causes, symptoms, diagnosis, and treatments for specific forms of arthritis.

- ▲ *Ankylosing Spondylitis*, No. 9050.
- ▲ *Arthritis and Inflammatory Bowel Disease*, No. 9062.
- ▲ *Arthritis in Children*, No. 4160.
- ▲ *Back Pain*, No. 4370.
- ▲ *Behcet's Syndrome*, No. 9065.
- ▲ *Bursitis, Tendinitis, & Localized Pain Syndromes*, No. 9055.
- ▲ *Carpal Tunnel Syndrome*, No. 9728.
- ▲ *Ehlers-Danlos Syndrome (EDS)*, No. 3428.
- ▲ *Fibromyalgia (Fibrositis)*, No. 4340.
- ▲ *Gout*, No. 4180.
- ▲ *Infectious Arthritis*, No. 4360.
- ▲ *Juvenile Dermatomyositis*, No. 9535.
- ▲ *Lyme Disease*, No. 4275.

- ▲ *The Marfan Syndrome*, No. 9338.
- ▲ *Osteoarthritis*, No. 4040.
- ▲ *Osteonecrosis*, No. 9337.
- ▲ *Paget's Disease*, No. 9064.
- ▲ *Polymyalgia Rheumatica*, No. 4330.
- ▲ *Polymyositis/Dermatomyositis*, No. 4390.
- ▲ *Pseudogout Syndrome*, No. 9054.
- ▲ *Pseudoxanthoma Elasticum*, No. 4080.
- ▲ *Psoriatic Arthritis*, No. 9053.
- ▲ *Raynaud's Phenomenon*, No. 9324.
- ▲ *Reflex Sympathetic Dystrophy Syndrome*, No. 5061.
- ▲ *Reiter's Syndrome*, No. 4350.
- ▲ *Rheumatoid Arthritis*, No. 4020.
- ▲ *Sarcoidosis*, No. 9057.
- ▲ *Scleroderma*, No. 9051.
- ▲ *Sjogren's Syndrome*, No. 9328.
- ▲ *Systemic Lupus Erythematosus*, No. 9052.
- ▲ *The Vasculitis*, No. 9056.

LEDERLE LABORATORIES *1-201-831-4692*
Public and Government Affairs
One Cyanamid Plaza
Wayne, NJ 07470

Publication

Questions and Answers About Rheumatoid Arthritis, an 11-page booklet about the forms of arthritis and the treatments.

NATIONAL INSTITUTE OF ARTHRITIS AND MUSCULOSKELETAL AND SKIN DISEASES (NIAMSD) INFORMATION CLEARINGHOUSE *1-301-496-2563*
National Institute of Health
Office of Clinical Center Communications
Building 10, Room 1C255
Bethesda, MD 20892

Publication

Arthritis, NIH Pub. No. 83-1945.

NATIONAL INSTITUTE OF ARTHRITIS AND MUSCULOSKELETAL AND SKIN DISEASES (NIAMSD) *1-301-496-8188*
Building 31, Room 4C05
Bethesda, MD 20892

Publications

Arthritis, NIH Pub. No. 83-1945.

Biennial Report of the Director, National Institute of Arthritis and Musculoskeletal and Skin Diseases NIAMS 1990.

NIAMS 1990: Arthritis, Rheumatic Diseases, and Related Diseases, and Related Disorders

Osteoporosis, NIH Pub. No. 89-2983.

Osteoporosis: Cause, Treatment, Prevention, NIH Pub. No. 86-2226.

Special Reports.

NATIONAL INSTITUTE ON AGING
Federal Building, Room 6C12
Bethesda, MD 20892

Publication

Osteoporosis: The Bone Thinner.

NATIONAL INSTITUTES OF HEALTH *1-301-496-2563*
Office of Clinical Center Communications
Building 10, Room 1C255
Bethesda, MD 20892

Publications

Arthritis, NIH Pub. No. 88-2982.

Arthritis Today, a videotape that can be borrowed.

ASBESTOS

The word "asbestos" comes from the Greek, meaning "inextinguishable." Workers exposed to high levels of asbestos in factories and shipyards and people who were exposed to air pollution containing asbestos have been shown to develop lung cancer, mesothelioma (a cancer of the lining of the chest and the abdominal cavity), and asbestosis (in which the lungs become scarred with fibrous tissue).

NATIONAL CANCER INSTITUTE (NCI)
Office of Cancer Communications
Building 31, Room 10A 24
Bethesda, Maryland 20892

Publication

Asbestos Exposure: What It Means, What to Do, a pamphlet that answers questions about such asbestos-related factors as risks, use of asbestos and potential exposure, detection and treatment of asbestos-related diseases, smoking, federal agencies concerned with the effects of asbestos exposure, and where to go for further information.

ASTHMA

See LungLine®, National Jewish Center for Immunology *under* Lungs

Asthma is a disease in which the airways may swell with mucus, blocking the flow of air into the lungs. Patients with asthma may react to factors in the environment which do not bother other people. In response to a trigger, the airways become narrowed and inflamed, resulting in wheezing and/or coughing. Reportedly the most common disease in this country, it afflicts about 5 percent of the population. Approximately 75 percent of those are children. Some 30 percent of all school absences—nearly 8 million days a year—are attributed to asthma. Approximately 2 million people with asthma suffer from limitations in activity due to their disease. Although asthma mortality in the United States is among the lowest in the world, reported mortality has been gradually increasing over the past ten years, especially in minority populations. The reasons for this are unclear, according to the National Asthma Education Program, but it is likely that a sizable proportion of the approximately 4,000 deaths per year that currently occur are preventable.

MOTHERS OF ASTHMATICS, INC.
See The National Allergy and Asthma Network/Mothers of Asthmatics *under* Allergy.

NATIONAL ASTHMA EDUCATION PROGRAM INFORMATION CENTER *1-301-951-3260*
4733 Bethesda Ave., Suite 530
Bethesda, MD 20814-4820

Publication

Check Your Asthma I.Q., NIH Pub. No. 90-1128, a 1-page handout that contains a quiz that gives general information on asthma in true/false format. The questions deal with such issues as whether asthma is considered a serious chronic disease, triggers of asthma episodes, early warning signs, medication, and exercise. Explanations are given for each question on the reverse side.

Facts About Asthma, NIH Pub. No. 2339, a 7-page pamphlet that combines illustrations and text to present the basic facts about asthma. The known triggers of asthma episodes are described, and the number of Americans diagnosed with asthma, the diagnosis of the disease, and the warning signs of an episode are addressed. There are suggestions for avoiding and lessening these episodes and exercise guidelines for the asthmatic. Current treatments and medications are discussed.

NATIONAL INSTITUTES OF HEALTH (NIH) *1-301-496-2563*
Office of Clinical Center Communications
Building 10, Room 1C255
Bethesda, MD 20892

Publication

Bronchial Asthma, a videotape that can be borrowed.

SCHERING-PLOUGH CORPORATION/KEY PHARMACEUTICALS *1-908-298-4000*
2000 Galloping Hill Road
Kenilworth, NJ 07033

Publications

Asthma and How to Live with It, presents an overview of asthma, what causes it, and what to do about it.

Asthma Therapy: Breathe Easier When You Know the Facts, addresses general questions concerning asthma and its treatment with theophylline.

A Brief Guide to Asthma, describes what triggers asthma and how to cope with it.

ATAXIA

The word "ataxia" comes from the Greek word *ataxis* meaning "without order" or "incoordination." Sometimes the word ataxia is used to describe symptoms associated with infections, injuries, or degenerative changes occurring within the central nervous system. Ataxia is due to a number of neurological disorders, causing slow, progressive deterioration of nerve cells in the spinal cord and cerebellum. Brain and peripheral nerves are frequently involved.

NATIONAL ATAXIA FOUNDATION *1-612-473-7666*
15500 Wayzata Boulevard, Room 750 *Fax: 1-612-473-9289*
Wayzata, MN 55391

Purpose To combat all types of hereditary ataxia. Services include providing information and referral to those affected by ataxia. Referrals are made to physicians or support groups when possible.

Publications

Ataxia Telangiectasia, defines A-T, symptoms, possible causes, and research.

Charcot-Marie-Tooth, fact sheet.

Essential Tremor, fact sheet.

Financial Planning, fact sheet on resources available for assistance and financial advice.

Frenkel's Exercises, exercise program that is designed for those with ataxia.

Friedrich's Ataxia, Fact sheet.

Hereditary Ataxia: The Facts, briefly describes the characteristics of recessive and dominant forms of ataxia.

ATOPIC DERMATITIS

See American Academy of Dermatology *under* Skin.

ATTENTION DEFICIT DISORDER

Attention deficit disorder, once caught in the catch-all basket of "brain damage" or "hyperactivity," is now generally agreed to be a neurologically based disorder. However, it is still not completely understood, and there is a great deal of research aimed at determining its cause or causes and its treatment. It generally involves poor regulation of attention, impulsivity, and motor activity. One afflicted, for example,

- Fidgets with hands or feet or squirms in seat.
- Is easily distracted.
- Has difficulty awaiting turns in games or group situations.
- Has difficulty following directions
- Has difficulty in sustaining attention in tasks or play activity
- Often engages in physically dangerous activities without considering possible consequences.
- Often talks incessantly.

CHILDREN WITH ATTENTION DEFICIT DISORDERS (CHADD) *1-305-587-3700*
499 N.W. 70th Ave., Suite 308
Plantation, FL 33317

Purpose CHADD is a nonprofit, parent-based organization formed to better the lives of individuals with attention deficit disorders and those who care for them. Through family support and advocacy, public and professional education, and encouragement of scientific research, CHADD works to ensure that those with attention deficit disorders reach their inherent potential. CHADD provides published literature for yearly membership, support group meetings, and free information packets for those who request information. Some chapters refer parents to professionals who are able to diagnose ADD.

Publications

ADD Fact Sheet.

Attention Deficit Disorders: A Guide for Teachers.

CHADD: Children with Attention Deficit Disorders, an 8-page brochure about attention deficit disorder and the organization.

C.H.A.D.D.E.R., a semiannual magazine.

C.H.A.D.D.E.R. Box, a monthly newsletter.

Medical Management Guide.

AUTISM

Autism is a syndrome of early childhood characterized by abnormal social relationships, language disorder with impaired understanding, rituals and compulsive behavior and uneven intellectual development. The ratio of afflicted males to females is 4 to 1.

AUTISM SOCIETY OF AMERICA — *1-301-565-0433*
8601 Georgia Ave., Suite 503
Silver Spring, MD 20910

Purpose The Society seeks to educate parents, professionals, and the public regarding autism, monitoring and advocating for legislation and regulation affecting support, education, training, research, and other services involving the welfare of individuals with autism. It provides information and referral to members, professionals, and the general public. The Society will refer to self-help groups and professionals who specialize in treating autism.

Publications

For members only.

COSAC-NEW JERSEY CENTER FOR OUTREACH AND SERVICES FOR THE AUTISM COMMUNITY — *1-609-895-0190*; *1-800-4AUTISM (in New Jersey only)*
123 Franklin Corner Road, Suite 215
Lawrenceville, NJ 08648

Purpose COSAC assists families, individuals, and agencies concerned with the welfare and education of children and adults with autism. COSAC is dedicated to promoting growth in services and providing a forum to develop and exchange information to benefit children and adults with autism. Provides information and referral, advocacy, short-term emergency care, speakers' bureau, parent education, professional education, support groups, and workshops. Refers to physicians, psychologists, dentists, diagnostic centers, and support groups.

Publications

Advocating for Your Child, a booklet about advocacy-related information geared for parents.

Autism: Basic Information, a booklet that gives an overview of the syndrome of autism.

Autism: Questions and Answers, a brochure for laypeople, it gives general facts.

Bibliography of Information for Professionals Serving Individuals with Autism and Severe Behavior Problems.

Checklist to Assess Service Appropriateness, a brochure.

Children Grow Up: Autism in Adolescents and Adults, a booklet with information about adults and adolescents.

Outreach, a newsletter.

Part One: Guidelines for Education & Treatment of Individuals with Autism, a brochure.

Part Two: Guidelines Pertaining to Adult Training/Workshops, a brochure.

Part Three: Guidelines Pertaining to Group Homes for Children and Adults with Autism, a brochure.

Practical Suggestions for Parents of Children with Autism, a booklet with articles on diverse topics.

12 Month Education for Your Child, a brochure that assists parents in getting an extended school year.

Understanding the Fragile X Syndrome, a brochure.

Update, a newsletter.

Numerous lists of suggested readings, schools, respite services, residential services, diagnostic centers and support groups.

In Spanish:

Autismo: Lo Que los Miembros de Familia Necesitan Saber, a booklet.

Autismo: Preguntas y Respuestas, a brochure.

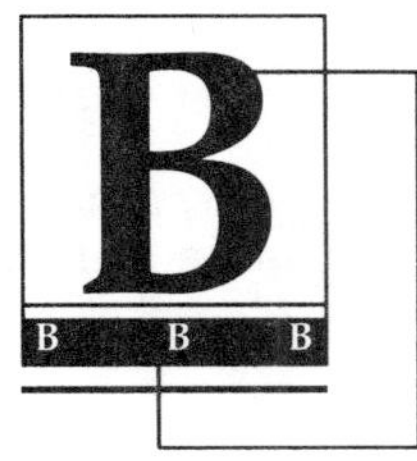

BABIES

Babies don't come with instructions. It may be difficult for a new parent to figure out the language of a newborn's cry and when a diaper change is required or the stomach is empty.

AMERICAN ACADEMY OF PEDIATRICS (AAP)
141 Northwest Point Rd.
P.O. Box 927
Elk Grove Village, IL 60007

Safe Sitter Program

The American Academy of Pediatrics approves of the Safe Sitter Program, which was started in 1980 by Patricia Keener, M.D., at the Community Hospital of Indianapolis after a friend's baby choked and died while with a baby sitter. Participants have a course in safety, emergency procedures, and general child care. They are provided with a detailed, easy-to-understand information packet to take with them on the job. For example, if a child is stung by a bee, the program instructs the sitter to "apply a cold, clean washcloth to the bee sting and to scrape, not pull, the stinger out with a fingernail. The sitter is also told to call a neighbor if the child has a rash or is pale, weak, or vomiting or to call 911 if the child has trouble breathing or has collapsed. The program also advises sitters not to watch scary movies that might make them afraid of normal house noises and to call their own parents to pick them up if the child's parents return home and appear to have been drinking. The program is now in five states and is being established in others. To find out if there is a program in your state or to help start one if there is not, write to the AAP.

FOOD AND DRUG ADMINISTRATION (FDA) *1-301-443-3170*
HFE-88
5600 Fishers Lane
Rockville, MD 20857

Publication

Feeding Baby: Nature and Nurture, Spanish version, FDA 91-2236S.

GERBER *1-800-GERBER 24 hours, including holidays*

Purpose *Baby Nutrition:* Trained operators will answer questions about how much and how often to feed infants and toddlers or when to start solid foods. They will not, however, answer medical questions.

NATIONAL HEART, LUNG, AND BLOOD INSTITUTE *1-301-496-4236*
Building 31, Room 4A21
Bethesda, MD 20892

Publication

Neonatal Respiratory Distress Syndrome (NHLBI Facts About), NIH Pub. No. 87-2893

NATIONAL INSTITUTE OF DENTAL RESEARCH (NIDR)
P.O. Box 54793
Washington, D.C. 20032

Publications

A Healthy Mouth for You and Your Baby, NIH Pub. No. 86-1255.

Prevent Baby Bottle Tooth Decay, a pamphlet advising how to avoid problems with baby bottles as far as teeth and weaning are concerned.

NATIONAL INSTITUTE OF MENTAL HEALTH (NIMH) *1-301-443-2403*
Information Resources and Inquiries Branch *Fax 1-301-443-0008*
Office of Scientific Information, Room 15C
5900 Fishers Lane, Room 15-105
Rockville, MD 20857

Publications

Pre-Term Babies. Caring About Kids Series, ADM 80-0972, 15 pages.

Stimulating Baby Senses. Caring About Kids Series, ADM 77-0481, 10 pages.

BACK TROUBLE

Back pain is one of the most common complaints of patients going to the doctor, with an estimated 80 million people in the United States suffering from some times of back ailment. The backbone consists of 30 bones called vertebrae. They are linked by strong ligaments and separated by flexible, flattened discs. Each disc is constructed of a fibrous outer covering wrapped around a jellylike inner substance. When you twist the wrong way or overstrain one part of the mechanism, it can cause a "back ache."

For back pain, *see* pages 30, 39, 66, 191, 231, 239, 311 and 312.

YMCA OF THE USA *1-312-977-0031*
National Director, Health and Physical Education *1-800-USA-YMCA*
101 North Wacker
Chicago, IL 60606

Purpose The National Council of Young Men's Christian Associations of the United States of America (the YMCA of the USA), which includes over 2,000 local YMCAs, is actively involved in improving spiritual, mental, and physical health. The national YMCA physical fitness and health program is based on preventive health care activities designed to head off heart disease, stroke, and other afflictions before they begin to develop. Prevention programs designed for people of all ages include fitness testing; aerobic conditioning; health education; individual and group fitness regimens; and behavior changing methods of weight control; smoking abatement; and stress management. Programs geared to children in kindergarten through grade 9 combine exercise with educational activities that teach cardiovascular health concepts. Prevention programs for adults offer fitness assessment and development of individualized programs for exercise and conditioning. Intervention programs include a program designed to prevent back pain and educational and rehabilitation programs for cardiac patients. Certification programs are offered for physical fitness specialists. The YMCA provides a variety of brochures dealing with such issues as physical fitness, risk factor education, and cardiac therapy. Flyers are published announcing new health programs.

BATTEN'S DISEASE
(Cerebral Sphingolipidosis, Late Juvenile Type)

Batten's disease is an inherited disorder of fat metabolism resulting in nerve tissue damage; skin pigmentation; bone lesions; and lumps found in the liver, spleen, lymph nodes, and bone marrow.

BATTEN'S DISEASE SUPPORT & RESEARCH *1-614-445-4161*
ASSOCIATION (BDSRA) *1-800-448-4570*
2600 Parsons Avenue *1-614-927-4298*
Columbus, OH 43207

Purpose The Association assists by providing information and emotional support to families of children with Batten's disease. It refers calls to other Batten disease families in their locale. Referrals are also made to physicians experienced in treating the condition.

Publication
List of BDSRA related articles, books, and video tapes.

NATIONAL INSTITUTE OF NEUROLOGICAL DISORDERS AND STROKE (NINDS)
P.O. Box 5801
Bethesda, MD 20824

1-301-496-5751
Fax 1-301-402-2186
1-800-352-9424

Publications

Friedreich's Ataxia, NIH Pub. No. 82-87.

Neurofibromatosis, NIH Pub. No. 83-2126.

Batten's Disease, NIH Pub. No. 87-2790.

BEHAVIOR

See also Health *and* Mental Health.

The lifestyle patterns and health behaviors, according to United States government researchers, are linked with major causes of morbidity and mortality in the United States today. Since 1981, the government has been conducting Behavioral Risk factor Surveys to help states obtain prevalence estimates of health behaviors that have been associated with risk of chronic diseases.

NATIONAL INSTITUTES OF HEALTH (NIH)
Office of Clinical Center Communications
Building 10, Room 1C255
Bethesda, MD 20892

1-301-496-2563

Publication

Behavior Patterns and Health, NIH Pub. No. 85-2682.

BEHCET'S SYNDROME

See under Arthritis.

BEREAVEMENT

See also Hospice.

A person whose loved one dies may at first be numb and then become stricken by intense grief. The pain usually starts to wane somewhat after six weeks and may be followed by depression and apathy. Emotional support is needed.

For loss of a pet, *see* University of Pennsylvania School of Veterinary Medicine *under* Mental Health.

AMEND (AIDING MOTHERS AND FATHERS EXPERIENCING NEONATAL DEATH) 1-314-487-7582
4324 Berrywich Terrace
St. Louis, MO 63128

Purpose AMEND is a free counseling service to parents who have experienced the loss of an infant through miscarriage, stillbirth, or neonatal death. One-on-one counseling to parents who experienced the death of their baby and educational services to the community are available. Referrals come to the organization through physicians or other medical staff. AMEND answers inquiries; provides advisory, counseling, reference, and current awareness services; conducts workshops and counselor training programs; distributes publications; makes referrals to other sources of information; and permits onsite use of collection.

Publications
Brochure.

Memorial Book.

Patterns of Grief in a Parent Experiencing Newborn Death.

COMPASSIONATE FRIENDS 1-708-990-0010
P.O. Box 3696
Oak Brook, IL 60522-3696

Purpose A mutual assistance self-help organization offering friendship and understanding to bereaved parents and siblings. There are over 600 chapters in the United States, and all parents are welcome to participate, whatever the age of their child who has died or the cause of death.

Publications
Brochure, a national newsletter, and a sibling newsletter are published quarterly. Books, brochures, videos, and other material are also available upon request. Since the organization is funded by voluntary donations and no dues are charged, a $1.00 donation would be appreciated to cover the cost of postage and handling.

BIOFEEDBACK

Biofeedback is a technique designed to reduce tension by the measuring biologic responses not normally felt or measured. When alerted by the signal to a change in pressure or body temperature, a person makes an effort to somehow produce more of the change. As a result, greater control over biologic responses is gained. It is used for

- Migraine headaches, tension headaches, and many other types of pain
- Disorders of the digestive system
- Blood pressure problems

- Heart beat abnormalities
- Raynaud's disease
- Epilepsy
- Paralysis and other movement disorders

ASSOCIATION FOR APPLIED PSYCHOPHYSIOLOGY AND BIOFEEDBACK
10200 West 44th Ave., Suite 304
Wheat Ridge, CO 80033
1-303-422-8436
Fax 1-303-422-8894

Purpose AAPB is the primary association for the study of biofeedback, self-regulation, and applied psychophysiology. The association, which has more than 2,300 members and 35 state chapters, exists to improve scientific, clinical, and educational applications in biofeedback and applied psychophysiology. Members of the association include psychologists, physicians, nurses, physical therapists, dentists, and students from the United States, United Kingdom, Europe, and Asia. Provides listings of biofeedback practitioners, researchers, and manufacturers of biofeedback-related services, information, and equipment.

Publication
Publications' catalog is available.

NEW JERSEY NEUROLOGICAL INSTITUTF®
MEMORY ENHANCEMENT CLINIC®
22 Old Short Hills Road
Livingston, NJ 07039
1-201-992-3300

Purpose Founded in 1976, New Jersey Neurological Institute® is a multidisciplinary group of professionals dedicated to aiding individuals who suffer from acute and chronic neurological problems.

Publications
Send a stamped, self-addressed, business-size envelope for
What Is Biofeedback?

BIRTH
See Childbirth.

BIRTH CONTROL
There are a number of reliable methods to avoid conception, each one with advantages

and disadvantages. The consensus among experts is: Oral contraceptives are 99 percent effective followed by the IUD which is 98 percent effective. Condoms plus spermicides are 97 percent effective as are the diaphragm plus spermicide. The condom and diaphragm alone are each 85 percent effective. The natural (rhythm method) is 25 percent effective.

INTERNATIONAL FEDERATION FOR FAMILY LIFE PROMOTION (IFFLP)
2009 N. 14th St., Suite 512
Arlington, VA 22201

1-703-516-0388
Telex 1-703-516-0391
Fax 1-703-516-0391

Purpose A nonprofit, public foundation, IFFLP provides leadership, guidance, and education in the field of family life education in general and natural family planning in particular; stimulates and assists in the formation of national natural family planning organizations in all countries; and facilitates communication among these organizations. Offers referral and technical assistance to not-for-profit services in more than 100 countries. Answers inquiries, provides consulting services, provides information on research in progress, conducts seminars, evaluates data, distributes publications, makes referrals to other sources of information, and permits onsite use of collection. Services are free, except for consultation, and are available to anyone, with priority given to members.

Publications
Pamphlets introducing IFFLP and its services.
Meeting proceedings.

NATIONAL INSTITUTE OF CHILD HEALTH AND HUMAN DEVELOPMENT (NICHHD)
Building 31, Room 2A32
Bethesda, MD 20892

1-301-496-5133

Publications
Facts About Oral Contraceptives.
Facts About Vasectomy Safety.

PLANNED PARENTHOOD FEDERATION OF AMERICA, INC.
Educational Resources Clearinghouse
Library and Information Network (LINK)
810 Seventh Ave.
New York, NY 10019

1-212-541-7800

Purpose The Federation promotes family planning, reproductive health, contraception, population, sexuality, and family life education programs and resources for professionals, parents, teachers, school students, teenagers, and other groups. It has a collection of materials on the areas just listed and in-house database. The Federation answers inquiries, provides information regarding programs and materials and research in progress for all areas of interest, distributes copies of some publications and data compilations, and makes referrals to other sources of information.

Publication
Newsletter, white papers, reference sheets, annotated bibliographies.

PLANNED PARENTHOOD OF METROPOLITAN WASHINGTON, D.C., INC. (PPMW)
Resource Center
1108 16th St., N.W.
Washington, D.C. 20036

1-202-347-8500 Ext. 221
1-202- 347-8500 Clinic

Purpose Funded by client fees, donations from the public, foundations, and grants, PPMW provides technical assistance and reference materials to staff, sex educators, professionals, and the general public in the field of family planning and human sexuality. It is interested in contraception, infertility, abortion, human reproduction, family planning, sexuality, sex education, religion and family planning, men's and women's health, AIDS, and STDs. It has a collection of 2,300 books, 150 films (16mm, VHS, slides), audiovisuals, curriculum guides, vertical files, and periodicals. And it answers inquiries; provides consulting, reference, and copying services; lends audiovisual materials; distributes brochures; makes referrals to other sources of information; permits onsite use of collection. Services are free, except for audiovisual materials and copying, and are available to anyone.

Publications
Free quarterly newsletter.

Men and Contraception: A Shared Responsibility, educators' handbook.

PPMW Agency Brochure, an overview of PPMW services.

BLADDER PROBLEMS
See under Urinary Tract.

BLINDNESS
See also Retinitis Pigmentosa.

The loss of sight is one of the most feared conditions. There is much that can be done to prevent it with early diagnosis and treatment. If you have any of the following signs or symptoms, consult an eye care specialist:

- Blurred vision not helped by corrective lenses
- Double vision
- Intermittent dimming of vision or sudden vision loss
- Red eye
- Eye pain
- Loss of side vision
- Halos around lights
- Crossed, turned, or wandering eye
- Twitching or shaking eye
- Flashes or streaks of light
- New floaters (spots, strings, or shadows)
- Discharge, crusting, or excessive tearing of eye
- Swelling of any part of the eye
- Bulging of one or both eyes
- Difference in the size of the eyes

AMERICAN FOUNDATION FOR THE BLIND (AFB) *1-212-620-2000*
15 W. 16th St. *1-800-232-5463*
New York, NY 10011 *1-212-620-2147 New York only*

Purpose The mission is to enable persons who are blind or visually impaired to achieve equality of access and opportunity that will ensure freedom of choice in their lives. AFB takes a national leadership role in the development and implementation of public policy and legislation, information and education programs, diversified products, and services. AFB serves as a national clearinghouse for information about blindness and visual impairment. It provides referrals to low-vision centers and publishes a catalog of low-vision aids; maintains regional offices throughout the country; and processes and makes available an identification card for all legally blind people that serves as a means of identification much as a driver's license does.

Publications

Publications' Catalog lists textbooks, periodicals, guides, manuals, research papers, public education materials, and general information publications on topics related to blindness and visual impairment.

Products for People with Vision Problems, a catalog featuring over 400 household, educational, and medical aids.

Video Catalog of 12 videotapes about blindness, visual impairment, and blind and visually impaired people.

BLIND CHILDREN'S CENTER *1-213-664-2153*
4120 Marathon Street *1-800-222-3566*
P.O. Box 29159 *1-800-222-3567 (in California only)*
Los Angeles, CA 90029-0159

Purpose The Blind Children's Center is a nonprofit organization that was founded in 1938. The Center provides diversified services to meet the needs of blind and partially sighted children, ages birth through 5, their parents, and siblings. Services include infant stimulation programs, preschool Programs, psychological support services, multihandicapped programs, and an educational correspondence program that has a toll-free number. The educational correspondence program provides access to information nationally; written correspondence serves families within and outside the United States. Inquiries are answered by child development specialists and educational consultants. Does not make medical referrals but does refer to services and parent support groups.

Publications

In both English and Spanish:

Dancing Cheek to Cheek.

Heart to Heart.

Learning to Play.

Move with Me.

Talk to Me I and II.

Booklets provide information that assists parents in understanding the dynamics of visual impairments and offer suggested activities parents and teachers can do with visually handicapped children.

LIONS CLUBS INTERNATIONAL — *1-708-571-5466*
300 22nd St. — *Fax 1-708-571-8890*
Oak Brook, IL 60521-8842

Publications

Age-Related Macular Degeneration, a pamphlet that describes macular degeneration and has a chart so that you can test your eyes to see if you may have the condition.

Aging and Sight Loss: Learning to Live Well with Limited Vision, a pamphlet about support groups and devices for the aged with limited vision.

Blindness, a pamphlet that describes the leading causes of blindness.

Cataracts, a pamphlet on what a cataract is and how it can be treated.

Sight Loss and Aging: Inevitable or Preventable, a pamphlet about early detection and treatment of vision disorders.

NATIONAL ASSOCIATION FOR THE VISUALLY HANDICAPPED (NAVH) — *1-212-889-3141*
22 W. 21st St.
New York, NY 10010

Purpose NAVH serves the partially sighted (not totally blind) with informative booklets, and large print loan library (free by mail); offers counsel and guidance to the partially seeing, their families, and the business community which employs them; and provides information and referral services. It also serves as consultant to the commercial publishers of large print material and acts as a clearinghouse for information about all services available to the partially sighted from public and private sources. Conducts self-help groups.

Publications

About Children's Eyes, small print. Informs about how to identify the child with visual problems and where to seek advice about children's eyes. Also available in Spanish.

About Children's Vision: A Guide for Parents, large print. Offers a better understanding of the normal and possible abnormal development of a child's eyesight.

Classification of Impaired Vision, small print. Describes various degrees of impaired vision.

Crochet Instructions (Granny Square), large print.

Daisies to Grow Indoors, large print. Gardening.

Diseases of the Macula, large print. Describes various conditions which affect the macular area and how to best maximize the use of residual peripheral vision.

Easy No-Work Perennials, large print. Gardening.

The Eye and Your Vision, large print. Information on common refractive errors and common eye diseases and general information on the human eye and how it works.

Family Guide: Growth and Development of the Partially Seeing Child, small print. Information for parents and guidelines in raising a partially seeing child.

Heartbreak of Being "A Little Bit Blind," small print. Summary of what it means to have impaired vision—with illustrations.

In Focus for Youth, large print. Newsletter issued at irregular intervals.

Knitting Instructions, large print for
- Baby blanket
- Full-length coat
- Ribbed pullover
- Topper-length coat
- V-neck sweater

Large Print Loan Library, large print. Listing of commercially published and NAVH large print books available through NAVH on a loan basis. Includes a limited selection of titles available for purchase.

List of Large Print Bibles and Religious Materials, large print.

List of Large Print Cookbooks, large print.

List of Large Print Crossword Puzzle Books, large print.

List of Low Vision Centers by State including Puerto Rico, large print. Specify state when you request this list.

List of Talking Book Distribution Centers by State, including Puerto Rico and Virgin Islands, large print. Specify state when you request this list.

A Patient's Guide to Visual Aids and Illumination, large print. Provides some practical principles, ideas, and an awareness of available devices that can be helpful in making the task of reading easier for the partially seeing.

Problems of the Partially Seeing, small print. Discussion of the meaning of being partially seeing and unique problems of these people; listing of steps NAVH is taking to ameliorate the problem, and activities for the young and adult partially seeing.

Seeing Clearly for Adults, large print. Newsletter issued at irregular intervals.

Visual Aids and Informational Material Catalog, large print. Descriptions and pictures of visual aids available from NAVH as well as some from commercial sources.

What Every Low Vision Patient Should Know, large print. Explodes some common myths about low vision. Also available in Spanish.

Brochures describing some of the commercially manufactured optical aids.

Brochures from commercial publishers of large print books; subscription forms for large-print editions of the *Reader's Digest Magazine* and condensed books, and *The New York Times* "Large Type Weekly."

List of articles in large print from the Federal Food and Drug Administration on health foods, nonprescription pain relievers, glaucoma, and so on.

NATIONAL LIBRARY SERVICE FOR BLIND AND PHYSICALLY HANDICAPPED
1-202-707-5100
1-800-424-8567
Library of Congress
1291 Taylor Street, N.W.
Washington, D.C. 20542

Purpose The Service provides free library service to individuals with visual impairments, offering braille and large print materials and recorded books and periodicals.

NATIONAL SOCIETY TO PREVENT BLINDNESS (NSPB)
1-708-843-2020
1-800-331-2020
500 E. Remington Road
Schaumburg, IL 60173

Purpose The Society is a nationwide volunteer organization of people helping people enjoy good sight for a lifetime. With a network of affiliates and divisions, NSPB works through research, professional and public education, and direct service programs to help eliminate preventable blindness. No referrals are made to physicians.

Publications

Single copies of up to two different brochures or fact sheets are free. *Do not* send a self-addressed stamped envelope.

Age-Related Macular Degeneration.

Amblyopia (Lazy Eye).

Battery-Related Eye Injuries.

Careful Use of Cosmetics.
Cataract.
Common Eye Problems.
Contact Lenses Choice to Improve Your Vision.
Diabetic Retinopathy.
First Aid for Eye Emergencies.
Floaters: Seeing Spots?
How's Your Vision? Family Home Eye Test.
LifeSight: Growing Older with Good Vision.
Play It Safe! (includes a safety checklist for your home).
Retinal Tears and Detachments.
Signs of Possible Eye Trouble in Adults.
Signs of Possible Eye Trouble in Children.
Strabismus (Crossed Eyes).
Sunglasses: Selecting the Right Protection for Your Eyes.
Understanding Dry Eye.
VDTs and Office Eye Issues.

SEEING EYE, INC. *1-201-539-4425*
Morristown, NJ 07963-0375 *Fax 1-201-539-0922*

Purpose The world's oldest dog guide school, Seeing Eye has placed more than 10,000 specially bred and trained dogs with blind people.

Publications

The "Bonnie" Book, a comic poster that children love.

The Guide, which gives the latest news on the organization and matters of interest to the blind.

If Blindness Occurs, which is useful for people who recently have become blind as a result of illness or accident.

Through the Motion Picture Service, P.O. Box 252, Livingston, NJ 07039, you can borrow free Seeing Eye films: *Meeting the Challenge of Blindness*, which shows the lives of four blind people and how each copes with the challenge, and *Harnessing Freedom*, the complete story of the Seeing Eye from its founding to the present.

VISIONS *1-212-477-3800*
817 Broadway, 11th floor
New York, NY 10003

Purpose Offers free services to anyone over age 55 with vision problems. Services include self-help study kits, counseling, professional support systems, consumer workshops, and an information center.

BLOOD DISORDERS

Blood is the fluid of life. It carries both nutrients and oxygen vital to fueling the body and it carries waste away from the tissues to help cleanse the body and regulate its temperature. Many things can go wrong with the blood supply including anemia, a decrease in red blood cells or oxygen carrying hemoglobin, to blood clotting or hemorrhage.

NATIONAL INSTITUTES OF HEALTH (NIH) — *1-301-496-2563*
Office of Clinical Center Communications
Building 10, Room 1C255
Bethesda, MD 20892

Publication
Blood Transfusion: Benefits and Risks.

BONES

See also under Calcium.

You have 206 bones that support your body or encase your vital organs. Your bones are alive. They are composed of living cells embedded in a hard structure of minerals with a soft center containing the marrow. The marrow manufactures blood cells.

AMERICAN ACADEMY OF ORTHOPAEDIC SURGEONS — *1-708-823-7186*
222 South Prospect Ave. — *1-800-346-AAOS*
Park Ridge, IL 60068-4058 — *Fax 1-708-823-8125*

BOTULINUM TOXIN

A substance released by the organism that causes botulism or severe food poisoning. It is being used to treat spasms of the eye and face. It has a paralytic effect. The peak of paralysis occurs five to seven days after it is injected.

NATIONAL INSTITUTE ON DEAFNESS AND — *1-301-496-7243*
OTHER COMMUNICATION DISORDERS (NIDOCD) — *1-301-402-0252 TDD*
Clearing House — *Fax 1-301-402-0018*
P.O. Box 37777
Washington, D.C. 20013-7777

Publication

Botulinum Toxin: A Consensus Statement, a 20-page booklet providing the opinion of experts on the use of the toxin for the treatment of crossed eyes and eyelid and facial spasms.

BRAIN

See also Alzheimer's, Aging, *and* Dyslexia.

The brain is the most important part of the nervous system—the captain of its organization. For the body to survive, the nervous system must be maintained. All other organs will undergo sacrifice to keep the brain going when under severe stress. The brain by weight alone is 90 percent of the central nervous system. One of the major functions of the central nervous system is communication—communication within its various parts and with the outside world. The signals that communicate information within the brain are electrical and chemical in nature.

NATIONAL INSTITUTES OF HEALTH (NIH) *1-301-496-2563*
Office of Clinical Center Communications
Building 10, Room 1C255
Bethesda, MD 20892

Publication

Brain in Aging and Dementia, NIH Pub. No. 83-2625.

BRAIN TUMOR

See also Arteriovenous Malformation.

A brain tumor is an abnormal growth caused by cells reproducing themselves in an uncontrolled manner. A benign brain tumor consists of harmless cells and has distinct boundaries. A malignant brain tumor is life threatening. It may be malignant because it consists of cancer cells, or it may be called malignant because of its location.

AMERICAN BRAIN TUMOR ASSOCIATION (ABTA) *1-312-286-5571*
3725 North Talman *Fax 1-312-549-5561*
Chicago, IL 60618 *1-800-286-5571 Patient/family hotline*

Purpose The ABTA distributes patient materials which discuss brain tumors and their treatment; funds brain tumor research; and refers to brain tumor support groups, treatment facilities, and other resource organizations.

Publications

About the Association for Brain Tumor Research, a brochure.

About Ependymoma, a brochure about tumors that arise from ependymal cells that form the central canal of the spinal cord and brain ventricles.

About Glioblastoma Multiforme and Malignant Astrocytoma, a brochure about the most common primary brain tumor.

About Medulloblastoma/PNET, a brochure that describes hope for this formerly hopeless type of brain tumor.

About Meningioma, a brochure about one of the most successfully treated brain tumors.

About Oligodendroglioma, a brochure about the slow growing nature of this brain tumor.

AFBTR Dictionary, a 39-page dictionary that explains medical terms patients are likely to hear or read.

Chemotherapy of Brain Tumors, a brochure that provides information on chemicals used to treat brain tumors.

Coping with a Brain Tumor, a 19-page booklet on treatments and the changes in the lives of those affected with brain tumors.

Immunotherapy of Brain Tumors, a 35-page booklet describing the therapy that involves stimulating the immune system.

Living with a Brain Tumor, a bibliography.

The Message Line, a newsletter.

A Primer of Brain Tumors: A Patient's Reference Manual, a 58-page booklet that provides information about diagnosis, treatment, and changes that a brain tumor patient may incur.

Radiation Therapy of Brain Tumors, a basic guide.

Radiation Therapy of Brain Tumors, a 27-page booklet on radiation therapy.

Shunts, a brochure about devices to reduce pressure caused by excess fluid.

When Your Child Is Ready to Return to School, a booklet that describes the cooperation required by an informed teacher.

NATIONAL INSTITUTE OF NEUROLOGICAL DISORDERS AND STROKE (NINDS) *1-301-496-5751*
Building 31, Room 8A06
Bethesda, MD 20892

Publication

Brain Tumors, NIH Pub. No. 82-504.

BREAST CANCER

See also Cancer.

One out of every eleven women in this country will develop breast cancer. By the time a breast cancer is felt, it has been in the breast roughly ten years and measures one third of an inch. Early diagnosis is instrumental in eradicating the cancer and the cause of death—it can mean a true reduction in mortality.

MY IMAGE AFTER BREAST CANCER
6000 Stevenson Ave., Suite 203
Alexandria, VA 22304

703-461-9595 Office
1-703-461-9616 Hotline

Purpose My Image is an information and support organization for women newly diagnosed with breast cancer or concerned about breast disease. A hotline is staffed by trained volunteers who have all experienced breast cancer. Volunteers do not offer opinions or advice on medical or surgical options, but provide current approved medical information. All conversations are confidential. Monthly Open Door Meetings present issues related to breast cancer by experts in their field. The goal of My Image is that "no woman face breast cancer alone.

Publications

A brochure about the organization.

NATIONAL ALLIANCE OF BREAST CANCER ORGANIZATIONS (NABCO)
1180 Avenue of the Americas
New York, NY 10036

212-719-0154 Answering machine

Purpose NABCO is a resource network established to provide written information to individuals interested in or wanting information on breast cancer. It provides written information and referrals and publishes a quarterly newsletter and a yearly resource list.

Publications

NABCO NEWS.
Resource List.
Various fact sheets pertaining to breast cancer.

REACH TO RECOVERY PROGRAM
c/o American Cancer Society
1599 Clifton Road, N.E.
Atlanta, GA 30329

1-404-320-3333
1-800-ACS-2345

Purpose The Reach to Recovery Program is a rehabilitation program for women who have had breast surgery. The Program, now established in American Cancer Society Divisions across the country, was begun in 1952 and integrated into the American Cancer Society in 1969. Reach to Recovery volunteers provide breast cancer patients with information on rehabilitative exercise, breast reconstruction, prostheses, and sources of prostheses. They also provide temporary breast forms to patients shortly after surgery. The program provides training for volunteers.

Y-ME NATIONAL ORGANIZATION FOR BREAST CANCER INFORMATION AND SUPPORT
18220 Harwood Avenue
Homewood, IL 60430

1-708-799-8228 24-hour hotline
1-800-221-2141
National hotline for United States and Canada, Weekdays 9 A.M. to 5 P.M. CST

Purpose Y-ME is a nonprofit organization that provides information and ongoing peer support to patients in all stages of breast disease. Founded in 1978 by two mastectomy patients, Y-ME services include a telephone hotline, one-on-one counseling, educational meetings, referrals, inservice programs for professionals, early detection workshops for the general public, and a wig and prostheses bank. Hotline callers are matched as closely as possible with volunteer counselors in type of cancer, treatment plan, age, and marital status. Pertinent literature is also mailed free of charge. The program answers general questions about breast cancer, treatment options, side effects, and general coping mechanisms and refers to physicians specializing in breast cancer treatment and to self-help groups. It also offers technical assistance to groups interested in establishing a program similar to the Y-ME program. Y-ME also conducts support meetings in nine states.

Publications

If You Thought About Breast Cancer, by Rose Kushner, distributed by Y-ME.

Y-ME brochure, lists services.

Y-ME HOTLINE Newsletter, reports the latest medical information on breast cancer.

BREAST FEEDING

Breast feeding has declined significantly in the United States over the last few years, according to a Tufts University study. Breast feeding helps babies' immune systems.

LA LECHE LEAGUE INTERNATIONAL
P.O. Box 1209
Franklin Park, IL 60131

1-708-455-7730
1-800-LA LECHE

Purpose A worldwide, nonprofit organization dedicated to helping mothers breastfeed their babies through education, information, encouragement, and mother-to-mother support. The free 800-line provides answers to mother's breastfeeding questions and/or referral to a local La Leche League group.

Publications
For a free catalog or information and promotional flyers available for international conferences, physicians' seminars, and lactation specialist workshops, call 1-800-LA LECHE.

BRONCHITIS

See under National Jewish Institute for Immunology and Respiratory Medicine.

BULEMIA

See Eating Disorders.

BURNS

Hot liquids, flames, electricity, vapors, chemicals, and sun's rays can all cause burns. The severity of a burn depends partly on the area of skin damaged and partly on the depth of the injury. A severe (third degree) burn will destroy all the layers of the skin, leaving a relatively painless area that may look white or charred.

NATIONAL BURN VICTIMS FOUNDATION (NBVF) *1-201-676-7700*
32-34 Scotland Rd.
Orange, NJ 07050

Purpose The Foundation is a nonprofit, publicly supported service agency based in New Jersey. Utilized nationally as a resource for information and referrals, the NBVF offers free professional services to New Jersey burn victims and their families. Besides taking an active role in burn prevention, care, and counsel, the NBVF shares its knowledge and expertise through educational and training programs presented to schools, fire departments, first aid squads, and community groups on burn awareness, emergency burn treatment, and preparedness for thermal disasters. It also makes referrals to physicians and self-help groups.

Publications
Brochure on the Foundation.
Charges for books and audiovisuals.

PHOENIX SOCIETY *1-215-946-BURN*
11 Rust Hill Rd. *1-800-888-BURN*
Levittown, PA 19056 *Fax 1-215-946-4788*

Purpose This worldwide organization provides peer support, counseling, and school and job reentry programs for burn survivors and families; refers to physicians specializing in burn treatments and to self-help groups; arranges probono surgery for burn survivors unable to pay; cooperates with American Red Cross at disasters involving burns, and offers scholarships to burn camps.

SHRINERS HOSPITAL REFERRAL LINE *1-813-281-0300*
2900 Rocky Point Drive
Tampa, FL 33607
Referral Lines: *1-800-237-5055 national hotline*
1-800-282-9161 (in Florida only)
1-800-361-7256 (in Canada only)

Purpose Shriners Hospitals provide treatment to save children's lives and restore their bodies to the highest level of usefulness. The hospitals conduct research into orthopaedic and burn care and train physicians and other medical professionals in the care and treatment of orthopaedic disabilities and burn injuries. The free telephone lines provide information about Shriners hospitals and the types of conditions treated. Parents can request an application for treatment through the 800 lines. Referrals are not made to physicians or self-help groups.

Publications

Burns, a brochure that describes the Shriners and their hospitals.

Combo, a brochure that describes the Shriners hospitals for orthopaedic and burn treatments.

Ortho, a brochure that lists orthopaedic Shriners hospitals.

20 Questions, provides facts and figures most commonly asked about the hospitals.

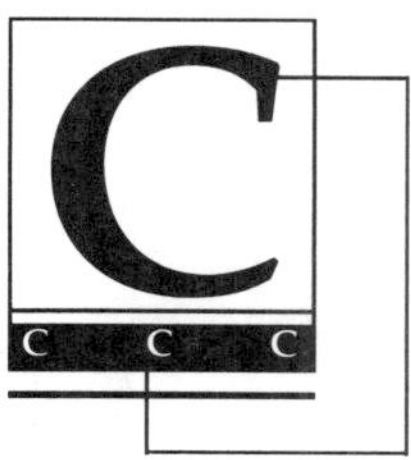

CALCIUM

The adult body contains about 3 pounds of calcium, 99 percent of which provides hardness for bones and teeth. Approximately one percent of calcium is distributed in body fluids where it is essential for normal cell activity. If the body does not get enough calcium from food, it steals the mineral from bones. Abnormal loss of calcium from bones weakens them and makes them porous or brittle and susceptible to fractures. Calcium deficiencies can result in osteopenia (less bone than normal, a condition preceding osteoporosis), and osteoporosis (a severe decrease in bone mass with diagnosable fractures) a condition that affects 25 percent of women after menopause. The percentage of calcium absorption declines progressively with age.

CALCIUM INFORMATION CENTER
New York Hospital-Cornell Medical Center
New York, NY 10021

Write to

Calcium Information Center
Box 907
Mt. Kisco, NY 10549
1-800-321-2681

Purpose The Center is funded, in part, by a grant from SmithKline Beecham Consumer Brands, makers of Tums®, and offers information on calcium. Barbara Levine, Ph.D., R.D., is director of the Center. She and her staff of nutritionists speak with concerned callers, giving advice on the telephone and sending booklets and nutrition information to callers by mail. The Center serves both the public and the medical communities.

CANCER

Cancer is not a single disease. It is the name of a group of diseases in which body cells go crazy and multiply without control. This can happen in any part of the body. More people are surviving cancer than ever before. For patients with cancers such as Hodgkin's Disease, testicular cancer, childhood leukemia, and many others, the picture is much more hopeful than it was a few years ago. Doctors know more than ever about how to fight cancer. Surgical techniques have improved. New drugs and other agents are working for many patients. Radiation treatment is stronger and more exact. And new combinations of treatments are giving better results. Cancer patients today may have a variety of choices about their treatment. Finding out that you have cancer and deciding what to do about it can be overwhelming. But having treatment choices helps you to feel more in control of the situation. You can even take part, if you wish, in new cancer treatments, and clinical trials, which may help you and/or other future cancer patients. If you have questions about what clinical trials are or any other questions about cancer, you may call

AMERICAN CANCER SOCIETY *1-404-320-3333*
National Office *1-800-ACS-2345 (within each state with a divisional office)*
1599 Clifton Rd., N.E. *1-800-422-6237*
Atlanta, GA 30329

Purpose More than 665,000 cancer patients a year are reached through the service and rehabilitation programs of the American Cancer Society. Specific information about cancer is provided as well as referral to Society services and other resources in the community to meet the social, psychological, and home care needs of cancer patients and their families. The program provides necessary, useful home care supplies and equipment. Volunteers drive patients to enable patients to maintain their medical and continuing care programs. *CanSurmount* is a short-term visitor program for cancer patients and their families. *Reach to Recovery* is the largest of the Society's patient-visitor programs. Laryngectomy rehabilitation is spearheaded by the International Association of Laryngectomees (IAL), a 275-club organization. Ostomy rehabilitation is a service that works with the United Ostomy Association. *Look Good . . . Feel Better*, a program in cooperation with the Cosmetic, Toiletry and Fragrance Association and the National Cosmetology Association, focuses on cosmetic techniques that can help people cope with body changes resulting from cancer treatment. The Society sponsors groups and individual education programs, distributes pamphlets and booklets, and provides audiovisual presentations for patients of all ages and their families to help them understand the complexities of the disease.

Publications

The American Cancer Society publishes several hundred brochures. You should request brochures according to specific cancer sites.

Cancer Facts and Figures is a comprehensive, 29-page booklet that is available to the public. It summarizes information about major cancer sites and services.

CANCER RESEARCH INSTITUTE *1-212-688-7515*
133 East 58th Street *1-800-99CANCER*
New York, NY 10022

Purpose The Cancer Research Institute was founded to foster the field of cancer immunology, which is based on the premise that the body's immune system can be mobilized against cancer. The Institute provides support in the form of fellowships, investigatorships, and grants to scientists engaged in research in the areas of cancer immunology and fundamental immunology. It also furnishes general information to cancer patients on how to get excellent care.

Publications

Cancer Research Institute HelpBook, an eight-step guide that informs patients about what to do if cancer strikes. It includes an extensive resource directory. *The book is free, but those requesting it are asked to send $2 per copy for postage and handling.*

Cancer and the Immune System: The Vital Connection, a booklet that answers commonly asked questions about cancer, the immune system, and emerging forms of immunotherapy.

FOOD AND DRUG ADMINISTRATION *1-301-443-3170*
HFE-88
5600 Fishers Lane
Rockville, MD 20857

Publication

Modern Diagnostics Help Detect Cancer Early, FDA 91-1173, reprint of *FDA Consumer* article.

LEDERLE LABORATORIES *1-201-831-4692*
Public and Government Affairs
One Cyanamid Plaza
Wayne, NJ 07470

Publication

Teamwork: The Cancer Patients Guide to Talking with Your Doctor, a 34-page booklet that covers what your doctor should know about you, what doctors wish their patients knew, and understanding and remembering what the doctor says and key questions to ask.

NATIONAL CANCER INSTITUTE (NCI)
Cancer Information Service
Office of Cancer Communication
Building 31, Room 10A24
9000 Rockville Pike
Bethesda, MD 20892

Hotlines:
1-800 4-CANCER
(in various states and regions)
1-800-524-1234 (Hawaii only)
1-800-638-6070 (Alaska only)

Publications

Write to or call

NIH Clinical Center
Building 10, Room 1C255
Bethesda, MD 20892
1-301-496-2563

For

Cancer and the Environment, a videotape that can be borrowed.

Cancer Treatment, NIH Pub. No. 84-1807.

Cancer, What Is It? a videotape that can be borrowed.

The Genetics of Cancer, NIH Pub. No. 90-3056.

NATIONAL CANCER INSTITUTE (NCI) *1-800-4 Cancer*
Office of Cancer Communications
Building 31, Room 10A24
Bethesda, MD 20892

Purpose Accurate, personalized answers to your cancer-related questions are only a phone call away. In Hawaii, on Oahu, call (808) 524-1234 (neighbor islands call collect). Spanish-speaking staff members are available to callers from the following areas (daytime hours only): California, Florida, Georgia, Illinois, New Jersey (area code 201), New York, and Texas. Cancer Information Service personnel will mail you free any of the publications listed here.

Publications

CANCER PREVENTION MATERIALS

Adjuvant Therapy: Facts for Women with Breast Cancer, a 10-page booklet that describes the drugs, treatment plan, side effects, and outlook for breast cancer patients receiving this form of treatment.

Advanced Cancer: Living Each Day, a 30-page booklet that addresses living with a terminal illness; discusses how to cope; and gives practical considerations for the patient, family, and friends.

After Breast Cancer: A Guide to Follow-up Care, a booklet for the woman who has completed treatment. Explains the importance of continuing breast self-examination, regular physical exams, possible signs of recurrence, and managing the physical and emotional side effects of having had breast cancer.

Breast Biopsy. What You Should Know, a booklet summarizing the biopsy procedures, what to expect in the hospital, awaiting the diagnosis, and coping with the possibility of breast cancer.

Breast Cancer Patient Education Series.

Breast Cancer: Understanding Treatment Options, a 20-page booklet summarizing the biopsy procedure, types of breast surgery (giving advantages and disadvantages for each), radiation therapy as primary treatment, and making treatment decisions.

Breast Reconstruction: A Matter of Choice, a 19-page booklet that discusses the techniques used in reconstructive breast surgery, possible complications, answers to common questions, criteria for choosing a plastic surgeon, and issues of emotional adjustment.

Chew or Snuff Is Real Bad Stuff, a brochure designed for 7th and 8th graders, it describes the health and social effects of using smokeless tobacco products. It features a fold-out poster.

Clearing the Air. A Guide to Quitting Smoking, a 24-page pamphlet, designed to help the smoker who wants to quit, that offers a variety of approaches to cessation.

Diet, Nutrition & Cancer Prevention: The Good News—Everything Doesn't Cause Cancer, a 16-page booklet that provides an overview of dietary guidelines that may assist individuals in reducing their risks for some cancers. Identifies certain foods to choose more often and others to choose less often in the context of a total health-promoting diet.

Good News, Better News, Best News . . . Cancer Prevention, a 16-page booklet that provides information on cancer risks and simple ways individuals can reduce their risks. Includes information on known and suspected risk factors, such as tobacco, diet, alcohol, and sunlight exposure, and describes specific actions people can take to reduce these risks.

Good News for Blacks About Cancer, a pamphlet providing brief information on ways black Americans can reduce their risks of cancer and detect cancer in its earliest stages.

Mastectomy: A Treatment for Breast Cancer, a 24-page booklet presenting information about the different types of breast surgery, what to expect in the hospital and during the recovery period, and coping with having breast surgery. Breast self-examination for mastectomy patients is also described.

Radiation Therapy: A Treatment for Early Stage Breast Cancer, a 20-page booklet discussing the treatment steps (surgery and radiation), possible side effects, precautions to take after treatment, and emotional adjustment to having breast cancer.

Why Do You Smoke? a pamphlet containing a self-test to determine why people smoke and suggests alternatives and substitutes that can help them stop.

PATIENT MATERIALS

Cancer Treatments: Consider the Possibilities, an easy-to-read brochure designed to make patients aware of clinical trials as a treatment option.

Chemotherapy and You: A Guide to Self-help During Treatment, a 64-page booklet, in question-and-answer format, that addresses problems and concerns of patients receiving chemotherapy. Emphasizes explanation and self-help. Includes glossary of terms and an entire section dealing with anticancer drugs and drug combinations.

Diet and Nutrition: A Resource for Parents of Children with Cancer, a 57-page booklet that contains information about the importance of nutrition, side effects of cancer and cancer treatment, ways to encourage your child to eat, and special diets.

Eating Hints: Recipes and Tips for Better Nutrition During Cancer Treatment, an 86-page cookbook-style booklet that includes recipes and suggestions for maintaining optimum, yet realistic, nutrition during treatment. All recipes have been tested. Originally produced by the Yale-New Haven Medical Center and reprinted by the NCI.

Help Yourself: Tips for Teenagers with Cancer, a 36-page magazine-style booklet that is designed to provide information and support to adolescents with cancer. Issues addressed include reactions to diagnosis, relationships with family and friends, school attendance, and body image. May be used in conjunction with audiotape. Produced in cooperation with Adria Laboratories, Inc.

Hospital Days, Treatment Ways, a 26-page hematology-oncology coloring book that helps orient the child with cancer to hospital and treatment procedures. Originally produced by the Ohio State University Comprehensive Cancer Center and Children's Hospital, Columbus, Ohio.

Managing Interleukin-2 Therapy, a 14-page booklet that explains what patients can expect during treatment, possible side effects, and management of these symptoms. Questions are included for patients to ask their health care providers while undergoing Interleukin-2 treatments.

Radiation Therapy and You: A Guide to Self-help During Treatment, a 42-page booklet that addresses concerns of patients receiving external and internal forms of radiation therapy. Emphasis is on explanation and self-help.

Taking Time: Support for People with Cancer and the People Who Care About Them, a 63-page sensitively written booklet for persons with cancer and their families that addresses the feelings and concerns of others in similar situations and how they have coped.

Talking with Your Child About Cancer, an 11-page booklet designed for the parent whose child has been recently diagnosed with cancer. Addresses the health-related concerns of young people of different ages and suggests ways to discuss disease-related issues.

What Are Clinical Trials All About? a 22-page booklet designed for patients who are considering taking part in research for cancer treatment. Explains clinical trials to patients in easy-to-understand terms and gives them information that will help them decide about participating. Includes a glossary.

When Cancer Recurs: Meeting the Challenge Again, a booklet detailing the different types of recurrence, types of treatment, and coping with cancer's return.

EARLY DETECTION MATERIALS

Breast Exams: What You Should Know, a pamphlet that provides answers to questions about breast cancer screening methods, including mammography, medical checkup, breast self-examination, and future technologies. Includes instructions for breast self-examination.

Questions & Answers About Breast Lumps, a pamphlet describing some of the most common noncancerous breast lumps and what can be done about them. Includes instructions for breast self-examination and a glossary of terms.

Smart Advice for Women 40 and Over: Have a Mammogram, a leaflet that discusses the benefits of regular mammograms for the early detection of breast cancer and presents breast cancer screening guidelines endorsed by NCI and 11 other leading medical organizations.

Testicular Self-examination, a pamphlet that contains information about risks and symptoms of testicular cancer and provides instructions on how to perform testicular self-examination.

When Someone in Your Family Has Cancer, a booklet written for young people whose parent or sibling has cancer. Includes sections on the disease, its treatment, and emotional concerns as well as a glossary.

Young People with Cancer: A Handbook for Parents, a 70-page booklet that discusses the most common types of childhood cancer, treatments and side effects, and issues that may arise when a child is diagnosed with cancer. Offers medical information and practical tips gathered from the experience of others. A glossary, bibliography, list of reading materials, and fold-out drug chart are included. Developed in cooperation with the Candlelighters Childhood Cancer Foundation.

GENERAL MATERIALS

Cancer Facts for People Over 50, a 4-page leaflet that contains facts about cancer, including signs to watch for, tests to have, and how to talk with a doctor about cancer.

Cancer Information Service Leaflet, a leaflet that explains the toll-free information system (1-800-4-CANCER), sponsored by the National Cancer Institute and regional cancer centers, to help the public obtain answers to their questions about cancer.

Did You as a Child or a Young Adult Have X-ray Treatments Involving Your Head or Neck? a leaflet that discusses the link between X-ray exposure to the head and neck and the possible development of thyroid tumors years later. Recommended examination and treatment for thyroid tumors are discussed.

Research Report Series:
- *Adult Kidney Cancer and Wilms' Tumor*, 25 pages.
- *Bone Marrow Transplantation*, 27 pages.
- *Cancer of the*
  - *Bladder*, 22 pages.
  - *Colon and Rectum*, 27 pages.
  - *Lung*, 23 pages.
  - *Ovary*, 18 pages.
  - *Pancreas*, 12 pages.
  - *Prostate*, 22 pages.
  - *Stomach*, 18 pages.
  - *Uterus*, 13 pages.

Hodgkin's Disease & the Non-Hodgkin's Lymphomas, 16 pages.
Leukemia, 20 pages.
Melanoma, 20 pages.
Mesothelioma, 10 pages.
Nonmelanoma Skin Cancers: Basal and Squamous Cell Carcinomas, 12 pages.
Oral Cancers, 18 pages.
Soft Tissue Sarcomas in Adults and Children, 20 pages.
Testicular Cancer, 19 pages.

Understanding the Immune System, a 36-page pamphlet that describes the complex network of specialized cells and organs that make up the human immune system. It explains how the system works to fight off disease caused by invading agents such as bacteria and viruses and how it sometimes malfunctions, resulting in a variety of diseases from allergies, to arthritis, to cancer. It was developed by the National Institute of Allergy and Infectious Diseases and printed by the NCI.

WHAT YOU NEED TO KNOW ABOUT CANCER SERIES:

Cancer
Bladder
Bone
Brain and Spinal Cord
Breast
Cervix
Colon and Rectum
Esophagus
Hodgkin's Disease
Kidney
Larynx
Leukemia, Adult
Leukemia, Childhood
Lung
Melanoma
Multiple Myeloma
Non-Hodgkin's Lymphoma
Oral
Ovary
Pancreas
Prostate
Skin
Stomach
Testis
Uterus

SPANISH LANGUAGE GENERAL MATERIALS

Buenas Noticias, Mejores Noticias, las Mejores Noticias . . . Prevencion del Cancer.
Guia Para Dejar de Fumar.
De Nina a Mujer.
La Prueba Pap.
Lo Que Usted Debe Saber Sobre el Cancer.

SPANISH LANGUAGE PATIENT MATERIALS

Anticancer Drug Sheets (in Spanish/English).
Boca (Mouth).
Colon y del Recto (Colon and Rectum).
Displasia (Dysplasia).
Estomago (Stomach).

Facts on Cancer Sites.
Prostata (Prostate).
Pulmon (Lung).
La Raditoterapia para el Cancer.
El Tratamiento de Quimtotetapia para el Cancer.
Utero (Uterus).

ANTICANCER DRUG INFORMATION SHEETS IN SPANISH/ENGLISH

These sheets on 30 of the most common anticancer drugs have been developed for Spanish-speaking cancer patients. Each sheet provides information about side effects, proper usage, and precautions. These sheets, a useful accompaniment to *Tratamiento de Quimoterapia para el Cancer,* were prepared by the United States Pharmacopeial Convention, Inc., for distribution by NCI.

Asparaginasa/Asparaginase
Bleomicina/Bleomycin
Busulfano/Busulfan
Carmustina/Carmustine
Clorambucilo/Chlorambucil
Cisplatin/Cisplatin
Ciclofosfamida/Cystarabine
Citarabina/Cytarabine
Dacarbazino/Dacarbazine
Dactinomicina/Dactinomycin
Daunorrubicina/Daunorubicin
Doxorrubicina/Doxorubicin
Estramustina/Estramustine
Floxiridina/Florxuridine
Fluorouracilo/Fluorouracil
Hidroxiurea/Hydroxyurea
Lomustina/Lomustine
Mecloretamina/Mechlorethamine
Melfalano/Melphalan
Mercaptopurina/Mercaptopurine
Metotrexato/Methotrexate
Mitomicina/Mitomycin
Mitotano/Mitotane
Plicamicina/Plicamycin
Prednisona/Prednisone
Procarbazina/Procarbazine
Estreptozocina/Streptozocin
Tamoxifeno/Tamoxifen
Vinblastina/Vinblastine
Vincristina/Vincristine

NATIONAL INSTITUTES OF HEALTH (NIH) *1-301-496-2563*
Office of Clinical Center Communications
Building 10, Room 1C255
Bethesda, MD 20892

Publication
Diet and Cancer Prevention, a videotape that can be borrowed.

CARPAL TUNNEL SYNDROME

See also under Arthritis and pages 29, 97, and 312.

This hand condition results from performing the same motions for hours at a time, as when computer terminal operators type continuously. The syndrome is named for the narrow tunnel in the wrist formed by ligament and bone. Tendons that enable the hand to close pass through the carpal tunnel. Injury to this part of the body can cause numbness or weakness, tingling and burning in the fingers and hands, or difficulty opening and closing hands. If the condition is not treated, permanent damage and loss of the use of the hand are possible.

AMERICAN PHYSICAL THERAPY ASSOCIATION
1111 North Fairfax St.
Alexandria, VA 22314

Publication
Send a stamped, self-addressed envelope for

Carpal Tunnel Syndrome and Posture and Back Problems Related to VDTS.

CEREBRAL PALSY

A complete or partial paralysis of the muscles—mainly of the limbs. It is not a single disease but a group of syndromes with a common denominator, some form of injury to the motor control center of the brain. The degree of the handicap varies from complete immobility to weak and poorly controlled movements.

AMERICAN SPEECH-LANGUAGE HEARING ASSOCIATION *1-301-897-5700*
10801 Rockville Pike *1-800-638-8255*
Rockville, MD 20852

Call or write for information on *cerebral palsy.*

NATIONAL INFORMATION CENTER FOR *1-703-893-6061*
CHILDREN AND YOUTHS WITH DISABILITIES *1-800-999-5599*
P.O. Box 1492 *1-703-893-8614 (TDD)*
Washington, D.C. 20013

Publication
Cerebral Palsy, F52.

NATIONAL INSTITUTE OF NEUROLOGICAL AND *1-301-496-5751*
COMMUNICATIVE DISORDERS AND STROKE (NINCDS) *1-800-352-9424*
P.O. Box 5801 *Fax 1-301-402-2186*
Bethesda, MD 20824

Publication
Cerebral Palsy, NIH Pub. 81-159.

UNITED CEREBRAL PALSY ASSOCIATIONS (UCPA) *1-212-268-6655*
7 Penn Plaza, Suite 804 *1-800-872-1827*
New York, NY 10001

Purpose There are 155 affiliates of UCPA nationwide that provide direct services to persons with cerebral palsy and similar disability. They conduct programs aimed at preventing cerebral palsy and helping those who already have the condition lead more productive and satisfying lives. Priorities of national UCPA include early intervention, employment, assistive technology, independent living, and family support. Will refer to self-help groups and physicians.

Publications

Family Support Bulletin.

The Networker.

Word from Washington.

CHARCOT-MARIE-TOOTH DISORDERS (CMT)

This is the most common inherited neurological disorder affecting an estimated 125,000 Americans. CMT is found worldwide, in all races and ethnic groups. CMT patients slowly lose normal use of their extremities as nerves degenerate. It is not a fatal disorder, and patients have a normal life expectancy.

CHARCOT-MARIE-TOOTH ASSOCIATION (CMTA) *1-215-499-7486*
Crozer Mills Enterprise Center
600 Upland Avenue
Upland, PA 19015

Purpose CMTA is organized to serve the Charcot-Marie-Tooth patients and their families and the medical community who treat the disorder. CMTA aims to increase the awareness of CMT and to foster research to find its cause and cure. The organization sponsors support groups, organizes regional CMT patient/family conferences, and holds professional CMT medical conferences.

Publications

CMT Brochure, a pamphlet briefly describing CMT, the CMTA, and how to obtain further information.

CMT Facts, a 16-page informational booklet.

CMTA Report, a quarterly newsletter.

CHARCOT-MARIE-TOOTH INTERNATIONAL
1 Springbank Dr.
St. Catharines
Ontario, Canada L2S2K1

1-416-687-3630
Weekdays 10 A.M. to 4 P.M.

Purpose A self-help organization run for and by people who have Charcot-Marie-Tooth disease, a progressively debilitating neuromuscular disorder. Provides information and referrals and answers questions. The director has the disease and is also the founder of the organization. Membership is by donation, no set fee.

Publications
Publications list.

CHILD ABUSE

See under Abuse.

CHILDBIRTH

There are many choices in giving birth today. Women may choose an obstetrician or a midwife, anesthesia or natural birth, home delivery or hospital delivery.

ASPO/LAMAZE (PSYCHOPROPHYLAXIS IN OBSTETRICS)
1101 Connecticut Ave., N.W., Suite 700
Washington, D.C. 20036

202-857-1128
1-800-368-4404

Purpose ASPO/Lamaze promotes optimal childbirth and early parenting experience for families through education, advocacy, and reform. Offers the 1-800 referral service for parents seeking ASPO-certified instructors and Lamaze classes throughout the country. Provides a national certification program for childbirth educators located in universities across North America.

DEPRESSION AFTER DELIVERY
P.O. Box 1282
Morrisville, PA 19067

1-215-295-3994
Answered by staff at various times during the week
1-800-944-4PPD
Answering machine that accepts incoming requests for packages of information

Purpose To provide support, education, information, and referral for women and families coping with blues, anxiety, depression, and/or psychosis associated with the arrival of a baby. Offers referrals to local support groups, telephone contacts, and professionals.

Publications
Publications' list.

NATIONAL INSTITUTE OF CHILD HEALTH AND HUMAN DEVELOPMENT (NICHHD) *1-301-496-5133*
Building 31, Room 2A32
Bethesda, MD 20892

Publications
Facts About Cesarean Childbirth.
Facts About Premature Birth.

CHILDREN

See also Infertility.

President Theodore Roosevelt said, "For unflagging interest and enjoyment, a household of children, if things go reasonably well, certainly all other forms of success and achievement lose their importance by comparison."

AMERICAN ACADEMY OF PEDIATRICS (AAP)
The Academy requests that you request information by mail, not by phone. Write to:
American Academy of Pediatrics
Department C
P.O. Box 927
Elk Grove Village, IL 60009-0927

Purpose The Academy has myriad brochures on several topics within child and adolescent health. One free copy of a brochure will be provided to you if you send a stamped, self-addressed, business-size envelope.

Publications
Brochures available are
AAP's Immunization Schedule.
Acne.
Alcohol.
Allergies in Children.
Asthma.
Avoiding Teen Pregnancy.
Bike Helmet Safety.
Breast Feeding.
Care of the Uncircumcised Penis.
Child Sexual Abuse.
Circumcision.
Choking Prevention and First Aid.
Cholesterol.

Cocaine.
Day Care.
Depression and Suicide.
Developmental Milestones.
Diaper Rash.
DPT Vaccine.
Family Health Insurance.
Feeding Kids Right Isn't Always Easy.
Fluoride and Dental Health.
Food Hassles.
Good Nutrition.
Growing Up Healthy Nutrition.
Healthy Foods.
Learning Disabilities.
Marijuana: Your Child & Drugs.
Sports and Your Child.
Sun Protection.
Teens Who Drink and Drive.
Television & the Family.
Temper Tantrums.
Tobacco Abuse.
Toilet Training.
You and Your Pediatrician.
Vaccination Q & A.

LEDERLE LABORATORIES *1-201-831-4692*
Public and Government Affairs
One Cyanamid Plaza
Wayne, NJ 07470

Publications

Otitis Media: A Children's Story . . . for Parents, a large, 23-page book that illustrates and explains for parents and children the causes and treatment of middle ear infections.

What You Should Know—And What You Can Do—About Haemophilus b Disease, a booklet that describes the cause of over half the cases of bacterial meningitis in children.

NATIONAL CENTER FOR RESEARCH RESOURCES (NCRR) *1-301-496-5545*
Westwood Building, Room 857
Bethesda, MD 20892

Publication

How Children Grow.

NATIONAL INSTITUTE OF CHILD HEALTH AND HUMAN DEVELOPMENT (NICHHD) *1-301-496-5133*
Building 31, Room 2A32
Bethesda, MD 20892

Publications

From Cells to Selves: The National Institute of Child Health and Human Development, NIH Pub. No. 89-83.

NATIONAL INSTITUTE OF MENTAL HEALTH (NIMH) *1-301-443-2403*
Information Resources and Inquires Branch *Fax 1-301-443-0008*
Office of Scientific Information, Room 15C
5900 Fishers Lane, Room 15-105
Rockville, MD 20857

Publications

Helping the Hyperactive Child. Caring About Kids Series, ADM 85-561, 9 pages.
Importance of Play. Caring About Kids Series, ADM 81-0969, 16 pages
Learning While Growing: Cognitive Development. Caring About Kids Series, ADM 81-1017, 14 pages.
Plain Talk About Adolescence, ADM 85-1065, 2 pages.

SINGLE MOTHERS BY CHOICE *1-212-988-0993*
P.O. Box 1642
Gracie Square Station
New York, NY 10028

Purpose Single Mothers by Choice is a national nonprofit organization founded in 1981 by Jane Mattes, a single mother by choice and a psychotherapist. The primary purpose is to provide support and information to single women who have chosen or who are considering single motherhood. There are members in nearly every state and in Canada.

Publications

Brochure.
Quarterly Newsletter.

CHILDREN WITH LEARNING DISABILITIES

See Learning Disabilities.

CHILD SAFETY

There are so many hazards both inside and outside the home to which active, curious, and innocent children may fall prey, it is a wonder any grow to adulthood. A number of childhood accidents can be prevented with proper precautions.

NATIONAL CHILD SAFETY COUNCIL *1-800-KID SAFE.*
Kid Safe Division
P.O. Box 1368
4065 Page Ave.
Jackson, MI 49204-1368

Accidents are the leading killer of children, making injury the number one health risk for children under the age of 15 years. The goal of the Kid Safe Project is to reach and educate as many children (and parents) as possible to reduce and, it is hoped, eliminate, this alarming trend. The *Kid Safe Project* is a free program for children age 4 to 14 and their parents. It is a division of the National Child Safety Council, a nonprofit organization dedicated to the safety of children through preventive education.

Publication
Kid Safe News

CHOLESTEROL

A blood cholesterol level of 240 mg/dl or greater is considered "high" blood cholesterol. If your blood cholesterol is 240 mg/dl or greater, you have more than twice the risk of heart disease as that of someone whose cholesterol is 200 mg/dl and you need to seek advice from a doctor who should conduct more tests. But, according to the National Heart Institute, a level of cholesterol of 200 mg/dl or more, even in the "borderline-high" category (200–239 mg/dl), increases your risk for heart disease. Levels less than 200 mg/dl put you at lower risk for heart disease. It does not mean "no" risk.

NATIONAL CHOLESTEROL EDUCATION PROGRAM *1-301-951-3260*
INFORMATION CENTER
4733 Bethesda Avenue, Suite 530
Bethesda, MD 20814-4820

Purpose The National Heart, Lung, and Blood Institute launched the National Cholesterol Education Program (NCEP) in 1985. The goal of the NCEP is to contribute to reducing illness and death from coronary heart disease by reducing high blood cholesterol.

Publications
Blood Cholesterol (NHLBI Facts About), NIH Pub. No. 90-2696, a 20-page fact sheet

that reflects newly released NCEP recommendations that healthy Americans should follow low-saturated-fat, low-cholesterol eating patterns to lower their blood cholesterol levels and thus reduce their risk of heart disease. Tips tell how to select and prepare foods lower in saturated fat and cholesterol and a chart gives saturated fat, total fat, and cholesterol levels for basic foods.

Dietary Guidelines for Americans: Avoid Too Much Fat, Saturated Fat and Cholesterol.

Eating to Lower Your Blood Cholesterol, NIH Pub. No. 89-2920, a 51-page booklet that explains the need to eat a diet reduced in saturated fat and dietary cholesterol to reduce elevated blood cholesterol levels. Contains tips on shopping for and preparing food. Also contains detailed appendices and a tear-out refrigerator poster of foods "to choose," "go easy on," and "to decrease" when following a blood cholesterol-lowering diet.

Even If You Are Feeling Like Superman, You Need to Know Your Cholesterol Number, poster encouraging people to have their blood cholesterol levels checked and to ask their doctor for the number.

Lower Your High Blood Cholesterol, NIH Pub. No 90-2972.

So You Have High Blood Cholesterol, NIH Pub. No. 89-2922, a 26-page booklet that describes the relationship of blood cholesterol to coronary heart disease, provides the cutpoints of "high," "borderline-high," and "desirable" blood cholesterol levels both in terms of total and LDL cholesterol, the factors that influence blood cholesterol levels, the difference between LDL and HDL, the role of diet and drug therapy, and how to monitor progress in a blood cholesterol lowering regimen.

CHRONIC FATIGUE SYNDROME (CFS)

Chronic fatigue syndrome, formerly called chronic Epstein-Barr virus syndrome, is a common and frequently debilitating illness, the cause or causes of which are still unknown. At this writing, the diagnosis of this illness is based on clinical observations, the particular constellation of symptoms and findings on physical examination. Laboratory evaluation may be suggestive of CFS and is helpful in ruling out other illnesses with similar symptoms. The following is the diagnostic criteria summarized by the Centers for Disease Control:

- Onset of persistent or relapsing fatigue with at least 50 percent reduction of activity level for at least six months
- Exclusion of other conditions by a physician and laboratory tests
- Six of the following 11 symptoms:
  1. Mild fever
  2. Sore throat
  3. Painful glands (lymph nodes)
  4. Muscle weakness
  5. Muscle pain
  6. Prolonged fatigue after exercise
  7. Headaches

8. Joint pain
9. Neuropsychologic complaints
10. Sleep disturbance
11. Acute onset of symptoms

- Two or three signs on physical examination
  1. Low-grade fever
  2. Throat inflammation
  3. Palpable or tender lymph nodes

NATIONAL CHRONIC FATIGUE SYNDROME ASSOCIATION *1-816-931-4777*
3521 Broadway, Suite 222
Kansas City, MO 64111

Purpose The Association is a nonprofit, voluntary organization formed to educate and inform the public, patients and their families, and health professionals about the nature and impact of chronic fatigue syndrome and related disorders, including chronic fatigue and immune dysfunction syndrome, chronic Epstein-Barr virus, and myalgic encephalomyelitis. Services include response to inquiries about the condition, educational and resource materials, and referrals to physicians and support groups. The organization also encourages legislative and private funding for research.

Publications
General information packet, which contains brochure on CFS, informational letter, membership application, and order form if other materials are desired (those are supplied at cost to cover expenses since it is an all-volunteer organization.)

NATIONAL INSTITUTES OF HEALTH (NIH) *1-301-496-2563*
Office of Clinical Center Communications
Building 10, Room 1C255
Bethesda, MD 20892

Publication
Chronic Fatigue Syndrome, NIH Pub. No. 90-3059.

CLEFT PALATE

Cleft palates, which may involve hard and soft palates in the mouth, occur once in 700 to 800 births. In severe cases of cleft palate, a special plate may have to be fitted on the roof of the baby's mouth before each feeding. An operation to repair the abnormality is carried out when the baby is older.

CLEFT PALATE FOUNDATION *1-412-481-1376*
1218 Grandview Avenue *1-800-24-CLEFT*
Pittsburgh, PA 15211

Purpose The Foundation seeks to educate and assist the public regarding cleft lip and palate (the nation's fourth most frequent birth defect) and other craniofacial anomalies and to encourage research in the field. The CLEFTLINE is a toll-free service providing information and referral to parents of newborns with clefts and other craniofacial anomalies and to adults with such defects. Referrals are made to cleft palate-craniofacial teams and to parent-patient support groups.

Publications
Numerous brochures and fact sheets available, including

The Child with Cleft Lip and Palate: The First Four Years, describes causes of clefting, most common treatment and therapies.

Feeding an Infant with a Cleft.

Genetics of Cleft Lip and Palate.

List of publications for sale.

COCAINE

See also Drug Abuse.

Coke. Crack. Coca. Nose Candy. Snow. It is derived from the leaves of the Coca plant cultivated widely in South America. Once widely used as a local anesthetic, it is still sometimes given for topical anesthesia in the mouth, throat and nose before surgery or other procedures. Because of its side-effects and potential for abuse, it has largely been replaced in medicine by safer local anesthetics. Cocaine is a central nervous system stimulant. Heavy regular use of cocaine can cause restlessness, anxiety, excitability, nausea, insomnia, and weight loss. Continued use may lead to increasing paranoia and psychosis. Repeated sniffing damages the lining of the nose and may eventually lead to the destruction of the structure separating the nostrils. People with heart disease, high blood pressure, and/or overactivity of the thyroid are at high risk of heart problems as a result of cocaine.

NATIONAL COCAINE HOTLINE *1-908-522-7032 Administrative office*
P.O. Box 100 *1-800-COCAINE*
Summit, NJ 07901 *24 hours, 7 days a week*

Purpose This is a free, confidential, national telephone helpline for people having problems with drug or alcohol abuse. The staff answer questions and give callers the names and phone numbers of treatment programs in the caller's local community. Some of the referrals on the list could include self-help groups or individual practitioners.

Publications

A brochure on the subject of cocaine abuse is available upon request from callers. The brochure provides some basic information about cocaine abuse in a question and answer format.

COCHLEAR IMPLANTS

The cochlea of the ear transforms sound vibrations into electrical signals for transmission to the brain along the auditory nerve. A person with a hearing impairment involving the cochlea can have a device implanted in the cochlea that picks up and sends sound vibrations.

NATIONAL INSTITUTE ON DEAFNESS AND OTHER COMMUNICATION DISORDERS (NIDOCD)
Clearing House
P.O. Box 37777
Washington, D.C. 20013-7777
1-301-496-7243
1-301-402-0252 TDD
Fax 1-301-402-0018

Publication

Cochlear Implants, a 10-page booklet on the benefits and side effects of implanted devices to aid hearing.

COLDS AND FLU

The words "common cold" and "flu" are ambiguous. They are often used to describe any one of a broad spectrum of complaints including a slightly stuffy, runny nose; an infection of the ears, nose and throat; an infection of bronchial tubes; or malaise, headache, cough and chest pains. In other words, the individual can be describing the symptoms of the common cold, bronchitis, influenza, or pneumonia. Most symptoms are caused by viruses but some symptoms may be caused by bacteria.

AMERICAN ACADEMY OF OTOLARYNGOLOGY HEAD AND NECK SURGERY (AAOHNS)
One Prince Street
Alexandria, VA 22314
1-703-836-4444
Fax 1-703-683-5100

Publication

Send a stamped, self-addressed envelope for

Antihistamines, Decongestants, and Cold Remedies.

Hay Fever Summer Colds & Allergies.

You and Your Stuffy Nose.

VICKS COLD BROCHURE
P.O. Box 15329
Stamford, CT 06901

Publication

Send a stamped, self-addressed business-size envelope for *Facts and Fallacies About Colds and Flu Transmission and Treatment Tips.*

CONTAGIOUS DISEASES

See Infectious Diseases.

COOLEY'S ANEMIA

Cooley's anemia is an inherited fatal genetic blood disorder. The medical names are thalassemia major and homozygous beta thalassemia. It is also commonly referred to as Mediterranean anemia. In the United States, Cooley's anemia strikes predominantly those of Mediterranean and Asian Indian heritage. The disease is found in 60 countries. Unless treated, children born with Cooley's anemia will die by age 3. The bone marrow of Cooley's anemia patients cannot produce enough hemoglobin (a component of the red blood cells).

COOLEY'S ANEMIA FOUNDATION
105 East 22nd St.
NY, NY 10010

1-800-221-3571 Staffed 9 A.M.–5 P.M. EST, with answering machine at other times
1-800-522-7222 (in New York only)
Fax 1-212-598-4892

Purpose The Foundation provides assistance locating physicians and treatment centers, insurance counseling, patient services, and scholarships.

Publications

All You Need to Know About Being a Carrier of Cooley's Anemia, about the thalassemia trait.

The Cooley's Anemia Foundation, Inc.

Lifeline Newsletter.

A Short Guide to the Management of Thalassemia.

Thalassemia: It's Your Choice, a brochure that explains thalassemia, an inherited condition.

What Is Thalassemia, an 84-page guide by Dr. Rino Vullo and Dr. Bernadette Modell designed to help thalassemics and their parents understand the disease, the reasons for treatment, and the hope for the future.

NATIONAL HEART, LUNG, AND BLOOD INSTITUTE (NHLBI) *1-301-496-4236*
Building 31, Room 4A21
Bethesda, MD 20892

Publication
Cooley's Anemia: Prevention Through Understanding, NIH Pub. No. 80-1269.

COSMETIC SURGERY
See under Plastic Surgery.

COSTS
See Health Insurance.

COUNSELING
See under Mental Health.

CREUTZFELDT-JAKOB DISEASE
A degenerative brain disease caused by a slow virus. It causes dementia, and loss of control of limbs and leads eventually to coma and death.

NATIONAL INSTITUTE OF NEUROLOGICAL DISORDERS AND STROKE (NINDS) *1-301-496-5751*
Building 31, Room 8A06
9000 Rockville Pike
Bethesda, MD 20892

Publication
Creutzfeldt-Jakob Disease, NIH Pub. No. 86-2760.

CROHN'S DISEASE AND ULCERATIVE COLITIS
Crohn's disease usually affects the small and large intestines, while ulcerative colitis strikes the large intestine (colon) and the rectum. Among the warning signs that should always demand a consultation with your physician:

- Persistent diarrhea

- Abdominal pain or cramps
- Blood passed through the rectum
- Fever and weight loss
- Joint pains; skin or eye irritations
- Delayed growth in children

CROHN'S DISEASE AND COLITIS FOUNDATION OF AMERICA, INC. *212-685-3440*
444 Park Avenue South, 11th floor *1-800-343-3637*
New York, NY 10016-7374

Purpose The Foundation maintains a coordinated national program of research to improve treatment and ultimately to find a cure; to educate patients, and their families, medical professionals, and the public through seminars, books, newsletters, brochures, medical forums, and public awareness programs; and to help patients and their families cope with Crohn's disease and ulcerative colitis through mutual support programs. Referrals are made to physicians and self-help groups.

Publications
Crohn's Disease, Ulcerative Colitis, and Your Child.
A Guide for Children and Teenagers to Crohn's Disease and Ulcerative Colitis.
Questions and Answers About Complications.
Questions and Answers About Crohn's Disease & Ulcerative Colitis.
Questions and Answers About Diet and Nutrition.
Questions and Answers About Surgery.

In Spanish:
Preguntas y Repuestas Acerca de la Enfermedad Crohn & Colitis Ulcerativa.

CULTS

See under Mental Health.

CUSHING'S SYNDROME

A number of abnormalities due to chronic overexcretion of cortisol and/or other hormones from the adrenal glands that lie above the kidneys. Among the classic signs are a "moon" face, poor wound healing, and skin that is thin and fragile.

NATIONAL INSTITUTE OF DIABETES AND DIGESTIVE AND KIDNEY DISEASES (NIDDKD) *1-301-499-3583*
Building 31, Room 9A04
Bethesda, MD 20892

Publication

Cushing's Syndrome, NIH Pub. No. 89-3007.

What to Do About the Flu (also available in Chinese).

CYSTIC FIBROSIS (CF)

See also under National Jewish Institute for Immunology and Respiratory Medicine *under* Lungs.

Cystic fibrosis, an inherited disease that causes lung and digestive problems, is usually fatal by age 30 years. It affects 1 in 2,500 Caucasian Americans; if both parents are carriers, their chances of having a child with CF are 1 in 4. Individuals currently can be tested for the six most common genetic mutations that cause 90 percent of the cases of cystic fibrosis. But the remaining 10 percent of cases are caused by any 1 of about 115 additional mutations, most extremely rare.

CYSTIC FIBROSIS FOUNDATION — *1-800-FIGHT CF*
6931 Arlington Road — *1-800-344-4823*
Bethesda, MD 20814

Purpose The Foundation raises funds to support research for new treatments and a cure for cystic fibrosis and provides public information and funds and accredits 120 CFF Care Centers nationwide.

Publications

Annual Report, summary of Foundation activity and finances.

CFF Home Health and Pharmacy Services, information on CFF home health services.

Commitment, biannual.

Consumer Fact Sheet, 4-88, "Public Assistance Programs"; 7-88, "Over-21 Programs"; 2-89, "Private Health Insurance."

Energy, Growth, and Cystic Fibrosis Nutrition Guide, McNeil Pharmaceutical.

An Introduction to Cystic Fibrosis for Patients and Families, a 95-page handbook easily understood by public. Gives information about CF.

Is an HMO Right for You? the CF consumer's 3-step guide.

Miscellaneous clips and updated material, as gathered.

Stop Paying High Prices, discount mail-order pharmacy flyer.

CYSTITIS

See under Urinary Tract.

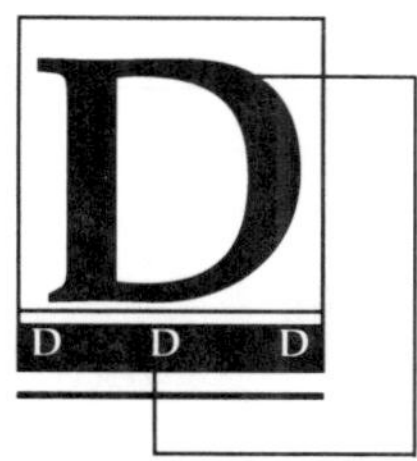

Dance

Dancing is a great way to express emotion, to exercise, and to become more coordinated and balanced. The movements of dance can also be healing. There are, however, strains and sprains that can affect dancers.

International Association for Dance Medicine and Science *1-612-831-4121*
4510 W. 77th St.
Edina, MN 55435

Purpose The Association provides a forum for all those working with dancers at all levels to help prevent injuries, obtain proper treatment for injuries suffered, and prolong dancers' careers. There is an annual scientific meeting for presentation by members. The Association does make referrals to physicians who specialize in the treatment of dance injuries.

Publication
Kinesiology and Medicine for Dance.

Deafness

There are two kinds of hearing loss:

1. Conductive hearing loss, caused by mechanical failure that keeps sounds from reaching the inner ear.
2. Sensorineural hearing loss, caused by nerve failure. Although sounds reach the inner ear, they are not perceived because the appropriate nerve impulses do not reach the brain.

Alexander Graham Bell Association for the Deaf *1-202-337-5220 Voice/TDD*
3417 Volta Pl., N.W.
Washington D.C., 20007

Purpose Founded in 1890 by Alexander Graham Bell, the organization has members in 35 countries. The nonprofit organization encourages hearing-impaired people to communicate by developing maximal use of residual hearing, speech reading, and speech and language skills. It promotes better public understanding of hearing loss in children and adults. The Association collaborates in research, works for better educational opportunities for hearing-impaired children, and disseminates information on hearing impairment, including its causes and options for remedial treatment. More than 20,000 inquiries are received each year from all over the world by mail, telephone, and teletypewriter relating to deafness. Questions are answered about tinnitus, cochlear implants, teacher training programs, oral interpreting services, lipreading courses, television captioning, and signaling devices for the home, to give just a few examples.

Publications

Programs and Services, an information sheet.

Publications Catalog, listing the books and products for sale by the organization.

Share in Alexander Graham Bell's Dream, a brochure about the organization.

DEAF COUNSELING ADVOCACY AND REFERRAL AGENCY (DCARA)
125 Parrot St.
San Leandro, CA 94577

1-510-895-2430 Voice/TDD
Fax: 1-510-895-5801

Purpose DCARA's goal is to enable hearing-impaired (deaf, hard-of-hearing, and deafened) people to live independent, productive lives, with full access to the services and opportunities available to the hearing population. To accomplish this, DCARA acts as a link between the deaf and hearing communities, providing the hearing community with information about deafness and related issues and providing the deaf community with access services and counseling. DCARA offices provide a variety of services to clients which include advocacy; counseling; interpreter referrals; independent living skills training; information and referral; job development, placement, and retention; community education and support groups; trades program; deafened adult program; and the DCARA bookstore. Clients served are individuals who are deaf or hard-of-hearing, and organizations and businesses that have hearing-impaired members or employees. Deaf/blind services available include training, personal needs, interpreters, and activities. The organization also has a Hispanic program and a senior citizens program.

Publications

DCARA News, a monthly newsletter.
Brochures.

DEAF-REACH
(FORMERLY NATIONAL HEALTH CARE FOUNDATION FOR THE DEAF)
3722 12th St., N.E.
Washington, D.C. 20017

1-202-832-6681

Purpose Deaf-REACH is a nonprofit organization, incorporated in 1972. Its mission is to maximize the self-sufficiency of deaf people needing special services by providing referral, education, advocacy, counseling, and housing. Through three group homes, two-day programs, and a walk-in community service center, Deaf-REACH annually benefits 150 deaf adults.

Publications

Agency newsletters and program brochures.

DOGS FOR THE DEAF

See New England Assistance Dog Service *under* Handicaps.

NATIONAL INSTITUTE ON DEAFNESS AND OTHER COMMUNICATION DISORDERS (NIDOCD) *1-301-496-7243, TDD 1-301-402-0252*

Building 31, Room 1B62

Bethesda, MD 20892

Purpose The National Institute on Deafness and Other Communication Disorders became the 13th Institute mandated by Congress within the National Institutes of Health in October 1988. NIDOCD conducts and supports research and training with respect to disorders of hearing and other communication processes, including diseases affecting hearing, balance, voice, speech, language, touch, taste, and smell, through a diversity of research performed in its own laboratories, a program of research grants, individual and institutional research training awards, career development awards, center grants, and contracts to public and private research institutions and organizations. The Institute also conducts and supports research and training through cooperation and collaboration with professional, commercial, voluntary, and philanthropic organizations concerned with research and training that is related to deafness and other communication disorders; disease prevention and health promotion; and the special biomedical and behavioral problems associated with people having communication impairments or disorders. NIDOCD supports efforts to create devices which substitute for lost and impaired sensory and communication functions and collects and disseminates information to health professionals, patients, industry, and the public on research findings in these areas.

Publications

About the National Institute on Deafness and Other Communication Disorders.

Cochlear Implants, Vol. 7, No. 2, May 1988.

Consensus Development Conference Statements.

General Information and Resources on Hearing, Balance, Smell, Taste, Voice, Speech and Language.

Hearing Loss, NIH Pub. No. 82-157.

Noise and Hearing Loss, Vol. 8, No. 1.

OCCUPATIONAL HEARING SERVICE
Dial a Hearing Screen Test
P.O. Box 1880
Media, PA 19063

1-800-222-EARS
1-800-345-EARS within Pennsylvania

TRIPOD GRAPEVINE
2901 North Keystone St.
Burbank, CA 91504

1-818-972-2080 Voice/TDD
1-800-352-8888 Voice/TDD
1-800-2TRIPOD (in California only) Voice/TDD
Fax: 818-972-2090

Purpose This private, nonprofit organization for hearing impaired children is committed to helping families raise and educate their deaf and hard-of-hearing children. The TRIPOD Grapevine is a national toll-free hotline offering up-to-date, unbiased consideration of and responses to the callers' concerns as well as two videotapes for parents and professionals. In the Los Angeles area, TRIPOD is a model private-public education program with many components—parent/infant, Montessori preschool/kindergarten, team-teaching elementary, and middle school classes. The TRIPOD programs serve children from birth through 6th grade in a fully integrated setting where deaf, hard-of-hearing, and hearing students, staff, and parents work cooperatively. Other components include family sign classes, day care, and a parent organization.

Publications

SENSE, a quarterly newsletter and videotapes for parents and professionals that are distributed nationally and internationally.

TRIPOD Is Something More, a brochure about the organization.

DEATH

See Hospice *and* Bereavement.

DENTAL IMPLANTS

See Teeth.

DENTISTRY

See also Teeth.

You may not smile when you have to go to the dentist, but the dentist can make your smile better. You should visit your dentist about every six months, not only to minimize tooth decay but also to check the health of your mouth. Your mouth may also reveal other health problems in your body.

AMERICAN ASSOCIATION OF ORTHODONTISTS
401 North Lindbergh Boulevard
St. Louis, MO 63141-7816

1-314-993-1700
1-800-222-9969
Fax 1-314-997-1745

Purpose The hotline provides consumers with a free 800 service to receive information regarding the benefits of orthodontics. After calling, the consumer receives appropriate information and a list of orthodontists in their area.

Publications

Adult Orthodontics: The Best Smile for Your Best Years, communicates that its never too late for braces. Answers questions adults commonly have.

Career Planning: Consider All the Angles—Orthodontics, presents a realistic view of what's involved in becoming an orthodontist as well as what you might expect from this career.

Elastics: Working Hard for Your Smile, provides tips on proper wear and care of elastics. Discusses their purpose in treatment.

Facts About Orthodontics: A Special Kind of Dentistry, answers common questions about orthodontics in a manner that patients of all ages can understand.

Good Beginnings: A Head Start for Healthy Smiles, contains great information for parents. Stresses the importance of early visits to family dentist and orthodontist. Points out problem areas that may indicate the need for orthodontics.

Next-to-Invisible: An Attractive Option in Braces, explains the benefits and shows examples of an attractive option in orthodontics for both children and adults—clear or tooth-colored braces.

Orthodontic Headgear: Important for Treatment, discusses the purpose and care of headgear, as well as safety precautions to follow while wearing headgear.

Orthodontics: More than Beautiful Smiles, an introductory brochure for new or prospective patients; answers typical questions patients have about orthodontic treatment.

The Psychological Benefits: Dr. Joyce Brothers on Orthodontic Treatment, presents the view that healthy, beautiful smiles are a boost to self-esteem, according to this noted psychologist and former orthodontic patient.

Removable Appliances: Are They Right for Your Smile? provides information on removable appliances, including why such appliances are sometimes necessary, tips on wearing and caring for removable appliances, and what types of removable appliances are available.

Retention: Hold That Smile, emphasizes the importance of this treatment phase and gives hints on caring for retainers.

Smiles, a patient newsletter printed quarterly. It is a poster-size publication filled with stories about brace wearers, tips about caring for braces, and more. The back side features a poster patients will want to keep. Mail newsletters to patients, hang them on your walls, or give them out at health fairs or school screenings.

Surgical Orthodontics: Profiles in Symmetry, contains questions and answers about reasons, risks, and rewards of this form of treatment.

Toothbrushing and Braces: Be Your Smile's Best Friend, highlights the importance of good oral hygiene and gives specific procedures for proper brushing while wearing braces.

NATIONAL INSTITUTE OF DENTAL RESEARCH *1-301-496-4261*
Building 31, Room 2C35
Bethesda, MD 20892

Purpose NIDR is the primary sponsor of dental research and related training in the United States. Its mission is to support studies to establish the causes, develop better treatments, and ultimately find ways to prevent or substantially lower the risk of developing oral disease. The NIDR covers 14 areas of oral health research:

1. Dental caries
2. Periodontal disease
3. Congenital craniofacial malformations
4. Acquired craniofacial defects
5. Dentofacial malrelations
6. Soft tissue disease
7. Craniofacial pain and sensory/motor dysfunction
8. Salivary glands and secretions
9. Mineralized tissues and fluoride studies
10. Pulp biology
11. Nutrition research
12. Behavioral studies
13. Implants, replants, and transplants
14. Restorative materials

Publications

The Extramural Program of the National Institute of Dental Research.

The Intramural Research Program of the National Institute of Dental Research.

The National Institute of Dental Research.

DEPRESSION

Depression has been called the common cold of mental illness. Most people feel depressed at one time or another. When someone is unable to rise from the depressed state and it interferes with the ability to lead a normal life, then professional help is necessary. Symptoms of depressive illness may include, in addition to feeling melancholy,

- Lethargy
- Poor appetite
- Trouble sleeping
- Disinterest in sex and other pleasurable activities
- Physical ailments such as headache and indigestion

NATIONAL INSTITUTE OF MENTAL HEALTH (NIMH) *1-301-443-2403*
Information Resources and Inquiries Branch *1-301-443-0008*
Office of Scientific Information, Room 15C
5900 Fishers Lane, Room 15-105
Rockville, MD 20857

Publications

Beating Depression: New Treatments Bring Success, OM 00-4053, 8 pages, reprinted from *U.S. News and World Report*, March 5 1990.

Bipolar Disorder: Manic Depressive Illness, ADM 90-1609, 6 pages.

D/ART Fact Sheet, ADM 90-1680, 2 pages.

Depression: It's a Disease and It Can Be Treated, OM 00-4028, 10 pages, reprinted from *Discover*, Vol. 7, No. 5, May 1986.

Depressive Illnesses: Treatments Bring New Hope, ADM 89-1491, 28 pages.

Helpful Facts About Depressive Disorders, ADM 89-1536, 8 pages.

Helping the Depressed Person Get Treatment, ADM 90-1675, 23 pages.

If You're Over 65 and Feeling Depressed... Treatment Brings New Hope, ADM 90-1653, 12 pages.

Let's Talk About Depression, ADM 91-1695, 2 pages, prepared especially for young blacks.

Plain Talk About Depression, ADM 90-1639, 4 pages.

What to do When a Friend Is Depressed: A Guide for Teenagers, OM 00-4036, 8 pages.

NATIONAL INSTITUTES OF HEALTH (NIH) *1-301-496-2563*
Office of Clinical Center Communications
Building 10, Room 1C255
Bethesda, MD 20892

Publication

Depression and Manic Depressive Illness.

DIABETES

Diabetes and diabetes complications are the third major cause of death in the United States. An estimated 14 million people in the United States have diabetes. Approximately 25 percent of people with diabetes have Type I, that is, are insulin dependent, whose bodies produce little or no insulin. Approximately 75 percent of people with diabetes have Type II, that is, are noninsulin dependent, whose bodies produce insulin but do not use it properly.

Signs and symptoms of diabetes are

- Weight loss or weight gain
- Frequent urination
- Excessive thirst
- Extreme hunger
- Fatigue for no apparent reason
- Blurred vision
- Frequent skin infections
- Slow healing
- Itching
- Nausea and vomiting

AMERICAN DIABETES ASSOCIATION (ADA) *1-703-549-1500*
National Center *1-800-232-3472*
1600 Duke Street
Alexandria, VA 22314

Purpose The Association strives to prevent and cure diabetes and to improve the lives of all people affected by diabetes. The ADA has more than 800 affiliates and chapters nationwide that provide education and other services to people with diabetes and their families, health care professionals, and the public. Local affiliates, which are listed in the White Pages of the telephone book, make physician referrals.

Publications

Diabetes.
Diabetes Care.
Diabetes Forecast.
Numerous public information pamphlets on various topics regarding diabetes.

JUVENILE DIABETES FOUNDATION (JDF) *1-800-JDF-CURE*
432 Park Ave. S., 16th floor *or 1-212-889-7575*
New York, NY 10016

Purpose The Foundation supports and funds research aimed at preventing diabetic complications and ultimately finding a cure. Referrals to physicians and self-help groups depend upon the policies of individual chapters.

Publications

A Child with Diabetes Is in Your Care.
Dental Care and Diabetes.
Diabetes and Kidney Disease.
Diabetes and Your Eyes.
Diabetes and Your Heart.
Diabetes and Nerve Disease.

Diet, Exercise, and Diabetes.
Dietary Management for Individual Diabetes: A General Guideline to Assist in Coping with the Dietary Requirements and Restrictions of Diabetes, stapled sheets.
Food Care and Diabetes.
Helping Research Find a Cure.
Information About Insulin.
JDF and You: The Search for a Cure.
Knowing the Warning Signs of Diabetes, a bookmark.
Living with Diabetes.
Low Blood Sugar Emergencies.
Monitoring Your Blood Sugar.
Oral Medications and Type II Diabetes.
Pregnancy and Diabetes.
What You Should Know About Diabetes.
Your Child Has Diabetes.

In Spanish:
Datos sobre la Diabetes, fact sheet.
Sepa las Senales de Advertencia de la Diabetes, a bookmark.

LIONS CLUBS INTERNATIONAL *1-708-571-5466*
300 22nd St. *Fax 1-708-571-8890*
Oak Brook, IL 60521-8842

Publications

Type I Insulin-Dependent Diabetes, a pamphlet that describes the causes and treatment of this condition.

Type II Non-Insulin Dependent Diabetes, defines the terms and treatment of this condition.

NATIONAL CENTER FOR RESEARCH RESOURCES (NCRR) *1-301-496-5545*
Westwood Building, Room 857
Bethesda, MD 20892

Publications

Family Behavior: Key to Managing Juvenile Diabetes.
National Diabetes Research Interchange.

NATIONAL INSTITUTE OF DENTAL RESEARCH (NIDR) *1-301-496-4261*
Building 31, Room 2C35
Bethesda, MD 20892

Publication
Dental Tips for Diabetics.

NATIONAL INSTITUTE OF DIABETES AND DIGESTIVE AND KIDNEY DISEASES (NIDDKD) *1-301-499-3583*
Building 31, Room 9A04
Bethesda, MD 10892

Publications

National Diabetes Information Clearing House
Box NDIC
9000 Rockville Pike
Bethesda, MD 20892
(Allow three to five weeks for delivery.)

Age Page: Dealing with Diabetes, DM-85, discusses Type I diabetes, including symptoms, detection, treatment, and self-help resources. Focuses on diabetes in older adults. Produced by the National Institute on Aging, National Institutes of Health.

Dental Tips for Diabetics, DM-16, a brochure for people with diabetes that discusses the relationship between diabetes and periodontal disease and describes symptoms of periodontal problems and preventive measures. Produced by the National Institute of Dental Research, National Institutes of Health. Also available in Spanish: *Consejos de Cuidada Dental para Diabeticos*, DM-108.

The Diabetes Dictionary, DM-84, an illustrated glossary of over 300 diabetes-related terms. The dictionary provides basic information for people who have diabetes and for their families and friends. Also available in Spanish: *Diccionario de Diabetes*, DM-02. Single copy free; additional copies 50 cents.

Diabetic Retinopathy, DM-20, discusses causes, development, and treatment of retinopathy as well as current research. Explains techniques (photocoagulation and vitrectomy) used to treat retinopathy and suggests resources for patients. Single copy only.

Insulin-Dependent Diabetes, DM-51, a booklet that explains diabetes and how it develops and describes the differences between the two major forms of diabetes, insulin dependent (Type I) and noninsulin dependent (Type II). Information about the diagnosis of insulin-dependent diabetes, its treatment, and the complications associated with it is provided. Treatment of diabetic emergencies is discussed, as well as recent advances in the management of insulin-dependent diabetes and current research on the disorder. Produced by the National Institute of Diabetes and Digestive and Kidney Diseases, National Institutes of Health. Single copy free; additional copies 50 cents each.

Monitoring Your Blood Sugar, J-09, brochure describing the purpose of and technique for self blood glucose monitoring. Includes information about equipment needed. Produced by the Juvenile Diabetes Foundation International. Single copy only.

Noninsulin-Dependent Diabetes, DM-81, a management guide for people with noninsulin-dependent diabetes. Includes chapters about symptoms and diagnosis of diabetes; diabetes management, including diet, oral drugs, and insulin; glucose monitoring; complications; and special situations and coping with diabetes. A list of resources is included. Single copy free; additional copies 50 cents each.

Periodontal Disease and Diabetes, A Guide for Patients, DM-21, an illustrated guide for people with diabetes discusses dental problems that may occur with diabetes and their prevention and treatment. Periodontal disease, which affects the gum tissue and bone structure that surrounds the teeth, can complicate diabetes management. The pamphlet describes how periodontal disease develops, its early stages, its relationship to diabetes, treatments, and the impact of periodontal disease on diabetes control. Preventive measures, including proper care of the teeth and gums and dental checkups, are described in detail. Produced by the National Institute of Dental Research, National Institutes of Health. Also available in Spanish: *Enfermedad Periodontal en los Diabeticos—Guia para los Pacientes,* DM-107.

Understanding Gestational Diabetes, DM-27, a 44-page booklet that is a guide for women who develop diabetes during pregnancy. It discusses symptoms and diagnosis of gestational diabetes, risk factors, tests during pregnancy, risks to and care of the newborn, and daily management including the use of insulin and blood glucose monitoring. Guidelines are provided for diet and exercise. The guide includes a glossary and sample forms for recording glucose tests and food and exercise information. Produced by the National Institute of Child Health and Human Development, National Institutes of Health. Single copy only.

NDIC Fact Sheets

Diabetes in Blacks, DM-113
Diabetes in Hispanics, DM-114
Diabetes Education, DM-115
Diabetic Neuropathy, DM-116
Diabetes-Related Programs for Black Americans: A Resource Guide, SM-44.

NATIONAL INSTITUTES OF HEALTH (NIH) *1-301-496-2563*
Office of Clinical Center Communications
Building 10, Room 1C255
Bethesda, MD 20892

Publication

Diabetes in Adults, NIH Pub. No. 90-3059.

SEVENTH-DAY ADVENTIST COMMUNITY HEALTH SERVICES *1-516-627-2210*
P.O. Box 1029
Manhasset, NY 11030

Publication

Possibilities for the Diabetic, description of the disease, with natural treatment options.

DIARRHEA

Diarrhea is abnormal frequency and liquidity of stools, which may be accompanied by cramps and a feeling of urgency. Causes include infections, irritation, inflammatory diseases of the bowel, toxins, certain medicines, or an overdose of laxatives. Nervousness and anxiety may also be a cause or contribute to the condition. Diarrhea can be life threatening.

NATIONAL ORAL REHYDRATION THERAPY PROJECT
2626 Pennsylvania Ave. N.W., Suite 301
Washington, D.C. 20037

Purpose The Project promotes a uniform, safe, and cost-effective approach to the management of diarrhea in the United States. The Project is guided by the leadership committee, which includes the American Academy of Pediatrics, the Association of Maternal and Child Health Programs, the National Association of WIC Directors, the International Child Health Foundation, the National Commission to Prevent Infant Mortality, and others.

Publications
Educational brochures parents (Spanish and English).
Educational brochures for health and medical professionals.

DIET

See also Food *and* Nutrition.

You may not have control over your heredity or your environment, but you do have control over what you eat. A great deal of information has been gathered within recent years about the benefits of reducing fat, sugar, and salt in your foods.

AMERICAN DIETETIC ASSOCIATION
See National Center for Nutrition.

AMERICAN SEAFOOD INSTITUTE — *1-800-EAT FISH*
Weekdays, 9 A.M. to 5 P.M. EST

Purpose The Institute is a trade association. It answers questions about buying, preparing, and storing seafood and will also address nutrition inquiries. It will not, however, answer questions regarding the safety of fish caught in specific waters.

AMERICAN SOCIETY OF BARIATRIC PHYSICIANS *1-303-779-4833*
5600 South Quebec, Suite 160D *Fax 1-303-779-4834*
Englewood, CO 80111-2210

Purpose The Society shares information among physicians interested in the treatment of obesity and other eating disorders. Dial-a-Tape is available to the public as well as referrals to physicians specializing in the treatment of obesity.

FOOD AND DRUG ADMINISTRATION (FDA) *1-301-443-3170*
HFE-88
5600 Fishers Lane
Rockville, MD 20857

Publications

Planning a Diet for a Healthy Heart, FDA 9102220, reprint of *FDA Consumer* article.

Sweetness Minus Calories Equals Controversy, FDA 91-2205, reprint of *FDA Consumer* article.

HCF FOUNDATION *1-800-727-4HCF*

Purpose A nonprofit foundation, High Carbohydrate Fiber, is run by Dr. James W. Anderson of the University of Kentucky, a fiber researcher. The phone line frequently deals with questions relating to diet and diabetes, cholesterol, heart disease, high blood pressure, and cancer. Caller can leave a recorded message at any time or speak to an operator, and a registered dietician will call back within 24 hours during business hours.

Publications

Newsletters and brochures.

INTERNATIONAL APPLE INSTITUTE *1-703-442-8850*
6707 Old Dominion Drive, Suite 320
McLean, VA 22101

Purpose The Institute is a trade association representing all aspects of the apple growing industry.

Publication

Send stamped, self-addressed envelope for

Delectably Nutritious Apples, which discusses the benefits of eating apples at all stages of life. Includes snack apple tips.

LONG JOHN SILVER'S, INC. *1-800-880-FISH*
101 Jerrico Drive
Lexington, KY 40579

Publication

Go Fish, tips on choosing fish and nutritive values of fish.

NATIONAL HEART, LUNG, AND BLOOD INSTITUTE (NHLBI) *1-301-951-3260*
Cardiovascular Disease Education Programs Information Center
4733 Bethesda Ave., Suite 530
Bethesda, MD 20814-4820

Publication

Check Your Weight and Heart Disease I.Q., NIH Pub. No. 3034, 2-pages; an 11-question, true/false quiz that addresses the independent relationship of obesity/overweight to coronary heart disease and its relationship to high blood pressure, high cholesterol, and smoking habits.

NATIONAL INSTITUTE OF DIABETES AND DIGESTIVE AND KIDNEY DISEASES (NIDDKD) *1-301-499-3583*
Building 31, Room 9A04
Bethesda, MD 20892

Publications

Obesity and Energy Metabolism, NIH Pub. No. 86-1805.

Peptic Ulcer, NIH Pub. No. 85-38.

NATIONAL INSTITUTES OF HEALTH (NIH) *1-301-496-2563*
Office of Clinical Center Communications
Building 10, Room 1C255
Bethesda, MD 20892

Publication

Obesity and Energy Metabolism, NIH Pub. No. 86-1805.

SARA LEE FREE & LIGHT LINE
Department MD
325 West Huron, Suite 315
Chicago, IL 60610

Publications

Send a stamped self-addressed envelope for
Free & Light Recipes.
Sara Lee Free & Light Fact Booklet.

SEVENTH-DAY ADVENTIST COMMUNITY HEALTH SERVICES 1-516-627-2210
P.O. Box 1029
Manhasset, NY 11030

Publications
Caffeine Questions, hints on kicking the caffeine habit.

Lose Weight Naturally, a 6-page pamphlet with hints about curbing overeating.

Naturally Tasty, a guide for good nutrition including vegetarian recipes.

USA RICE COUNCIL 1-713-270-6699
P.O. Box 740121
Houston, TX 77274

Purpose To promote U.S.-grown rice.

Publications
Send a stamped, self-addressed, envelope for

Light, Lean & Low Fat, recipes low in fat.

SportSense, a guide to good eating and exercise habits plus healthful recipes.

DIGESTIVE PROBLEMS

See also Crohn's *and* Colitis Foundation of America, Inc.

There are a lot of parts to your digestive system as you probably learned whenever it became upset. Functional disorders include painful, difficult, or disturbed digestion causing some combination of nausea, regurgitation, vomiting, heartburn, bloating, and abdominal pain or fullness. Irritable bowel syndrome is an intestinal disorder characterized by gas, abdominal pain, and diarrhea and/or constipation. Ulcers, pancreatitis, liver disorders, gallbladder trouble, and mouth and esophageal problems may all be considered digestive problems. Easy to "swallow" medical information is available for all those conditions.

AMERICAN SOCIETY FOR GASTROINTESTINAL ENDOSCOPY
13 Elm Street
Manchester, MA 01944

Purpose The Society provides information, training, and practice guidelines on gastrointestinal endoscopic techniques.

Publications
Patient information brochures.

DIGESTIVE DISEASE NATIONAL COALITION (DDNC) *1-202-544-7497*
711 Second Street N.E., Suite 200 *Fax 1-202-546-7105*
Washington, D.C. 20002

Purpose The objective of the DDNC is to increase public awareness about digestive diseases, provide educational material, and support federal funding of digestive disease research. Educational brochures are distributed and referrals are made to DDNC member organizations.

Publications

Help for Heartburn.
Help for Heartburn: Favorite Gourmet Recipes from Around the World.
When You Suffer the Pain and Discomfort of Digestive Diseases.
Your Gallstones: Diagnosis and Treatment.

NATIONAL DIGESTIVE DISEASES INFORMATION CLEARINGHOUSE *1-301-468-6344*
Box NDDIC
Bethesda, MD 20892

Publications

Bleeding in the Digestive Tract, NIH Pub. No. 89-1133.
Diagnostic Tests for Digestive Diseases: X-rays and Ultrasound, NIH Pub. No. 87-887.
Diarrhea: Infectious and Other Causes, NIH Pub. No. 86-2749.
Digestive Diseases Annotated Listing of Patient Education Materials, NIH Pub. No. 87-2906.
Digestive Health and Disease: A Glossary, NIH Pub. No. 86-2750.
Diverticulosis and Diverticulitis, NIH Pub. No. 90-1163.
Facts and Fallacies About Digestive Diseases, NIH Pub. No. 86-2673.

PATIENT INFORMATION PAMPHLETS

About Stomach Ulcers (64).
Age Page: Constipation (36).
Age Page: Nutrition-A Life-Long Concern (39).
Cirrhosis of the Liver (73).
Diagnostic Tests for Digestive Diseases: X-rays and Ultrasound (7).
Digestive Health and Disease: A Glossary (1).
Facts & Fallacies About Digestive Diseases (2).
Gallstones (97).
Gas in the Digestive Tract (30).
Heartburn (26).
Hemorrhoids (59).
IBD and IBS: Two Very Different Problems (13).

Inflammatory Bowel Disease (9).
Irritable Bowel Syndrome (14).
Lactose Intolerance (48).
Peptic Ulcers (65).
Smoking and Your Digestive System (52).
Ulcerative Colitis (15).
What Is Constipation? (35).
What Is Dyspepsia? (50).
What Is Hiatal Hernia? (31).
What Is Pancreatitis? (71).
Your Digestive System and How It Works (3).

NATIONAL INSTITUTE OF DIABETES AND DIGESTIVE AND KIDNEY DISEASES (NIDDKD)
NIH Clinical Center
Building 10, Room 1C255L
Bethesda, MD 20892

1-301-496-3583
1-301-496-2563

Publication

Obesity and Energy Metabolism, NIH Pub. No. 86-1805.

DISABILITIES

The National Center on Health Statistics estimates that over 18 million Americans experience hearing losses. Hearing impairment affects more Americans than any other physical disability. The Center estimates that over 15 million people in the United States are visually impaired.

Mobility impairments limit the capacity of individuals to walk freely. This includes people who have difficulty walking long distances or climbing stairs or who use wheelchairs. The following conditions are among those that may cause a person to be mobility impaired: cancer, arthritis, amputation, cerebral palsy, multiple sclerosis, polio, spinal cord injury, stroke, or head injury. Neuromuscular conditions such as multiple sclerosis and cerebral palsy, paralysis of hands and arms caused by spinal cord injury, the effects of medication, and a variety of other conditions, including cumulative trauma disorders such as carpal tunnel syndrome, may cause difficulty in performing such manual tasks as using the fingers and hands for gripping, typing, opening drawers, use of arms and hands for reaching, or use of the sensation of touch. For some individuals, lifting may cause fainting, dizziness, or seizures. In other words, disabilities are very common. Some create more challenges to the people that have them than others. The Americans with Disabilities Act was signed by President George Bush, July 26, 1990. It opened the way for many more people with disabilities who are properly trained and qualified to obtain employment. The organizations listed here help those physically challenged and their families to obtain information that will enable those with disabilities to make the most of their abilities.

ADVOCACY CENTER FOR THE ELDERLY AND DISABLED*
210 O'Keefe Ave., Suite 700
New Orleans, LA 70112

1-800-662-7705 (Louisiana only)

ERIC CLEARINGHOUSE ON HANDICAPPED AND GIFTED CHILDREN*
The Council for Exceptional Children
1920 Association Drive
Reston, VA 22091

1-703-620-3660 Voice/TDD
1-703-620-3660

HEATH RESOURCE CENTER*
Higher Education and Adult Training for People with Disabilities Resource Center
1 Dupont Circle, N.W., Suite 800
Washington, D.C. 20036-1193

1-800-544-3284
1-202-939-9320 Voice/TDD

IBM NATIONAL SUPPORT CENTER FOR PERSONS WITH DISABILITIES*
P.O. Box 2150
Atlanta, GA 30055

1-800-426-2133
1-404-238-4806 TDD

Purpose Center provides information about the aid computers can offer people with vision, hearing, speech, learning, mental retardation, and mobility problems. Assistive devices and software services available.

INSTITUTE OF LOGOPEDICS*
2400 Jardine Dr.
Wichita, KS 67219

1-316-262-8271
1-800-835-1043
1-800-937-4644

Purpose The Institute is a residential school offering special education to children ages 3–21 years with multiple disabilities. Children live in a homelike environment and attend classes on a 40-acre campus. Callers receive referrals to other programs, evaluation and diagnostic facilities, physicians, and parent organizations available in their area.

Publications

Life Contributions, a videotape showing the Residential School is available to interested parents and agencies.

Residential School Viewbook, describes the Institute program.

*A federally supported clearinghouse related to disabilities.

JAN (JOB ACCOMMODATION NETWORK)
West Virginia University
809 Allen Hall
P.O. Box 6123
Morgantown, WV 26506-6123

1-800-JAN-7234
(in the United States only)
1-800-JAN-CANA (in Canada only)
1-800-DIAL-JAN Computer/modem

Purpose An international information network and consulting resource for accommodating persons with disabilities in the workplace. Offers help to employees who need some assistance to stay on the job and to employers interviewing an individual with a disability or trying to make a business accessible to all customers. JAN is a service of the President's Committee on Employment of People with Disabilities. There is no charge for the service.

Publication
Brochure about JAN.

NATIONAL CENTER FOR YOUTH WITH DISABILITIES (NCYD)*
University of Minnesota
Box 721-UMHC
Harvard Street at East River Road
Minneapolis, MN 55455

1-612-626-2825
1-800-333-6293
1-612-624-3939 TDD

Purpose NCYD is an information and resource center focusing on adolescents with chronic illnesses and disabilities and the issues surrounding their transition to adult life. NCYD maintains the National Resource Library, a computerized database containing current information about youth with disabilities. No referrals to physicians, but referrals are made to parent support groups or other appropriate disability related programs.

Publications
Connections, a newsletter.

CYDLINE Reviews, a series of annotated bibliographies.

FYI Bulletin, a series of fact sheets.

National Center for Youth with Disabilities, a brochure on the information and resource center.

National Resource Library on Youth with Disabilities, a brochure describing NCYD's computerized database.

Youth with Disabilities Publications List, a list of publications for sale.

NATIONAL CRISTINA FOUNDATION (NCF)*
42 Hillcrest Drive
Pelham Manor, NY 10803

1-914-738-7494
1-800-CRISTINA
Fax 1-914-738-1571

*A federally supported clearinghouse related to disabilities.

Purpose This nonprofit foundation's goal is to share computer and high technology applications to help people in need lead productive lives. Donations of used and surplus, earlier-generation computers and related technology are directed through NCF to partner organizations in the NCF network. These organizations adapt the machines to the special needs of people with disabilities and other special needs. The disabled, at risk students, and the disadvantaged are trained to develop skills needed for employment.

Publication
Your Old Computer Has the Power to Give New Life, a brochure.

NATIONAL EASTER SEAL SOCIETY* — *1-312-726-6200*
70 E. Lake Street — *1-312-726-4258 TDD*
Chicago, IL 60601

Purpose The Society helps people with disabilities to achieve maximum independence. It provides rehabilitation therapy, technological assistance, camping and recreational services, prevention and screening, advocacy, and public education. Referrals to physicians and self-help groups are made through local Easter Seal societies.

Publications
Publications' catalog.

NATIONAL INFORMATION CENTER FOR CHILDREN AND YOUTHS WITH DISABILITIES (NICCYD)* — *1-703-893-6061*, *1-800-999-5599*, *1-703-893-8614 TDD*
P.O. Box 1492
Washington, D.C. 20013 (mailing address)
7926 Jones Branch Dr., Suite 1100
McLean, VA 22101 (street address)

Purpose NICCYD provides free information to assist parents, educators, caregivers, advocates, and others in helping children and youth with disabilities become participating members of the community. Personnel answer specific questions, refer callers to other organizations and sources of help, send prepared information packets and publications on current issues, and provide technical assistance to parents and professional groups.

Publications

NICHCY News Digest, an 8- to 12-page newsletter published three times a year and covering one topic in depth in each issue.

Transition Summary, an 8- to 12-page newsletter published annually, covering one topic in depth each issue, for youth moving out of high school to work, college, and independent living.

*A federally supported clearinghouse related to disabilities.

GENERAL RESOURCE

Brochure, GR-1.
General Information about Disabilities, GR-3.
List of National Resources, GR-2.
National Toll Free Numbers, GR-5.
Public Agencies Fact Sheet, GR-4.
Publications list, GR-8.
State Resource Sheet: State, GR-6.

NEWS DIGEST

Alternatives for Community Living, ND-4.
Assistive Technology: Becoming an Informed Consumer, ND-13.
Children with Disabilities: Understanding Sibling Issues, ND-11.
Early Intervention for Children Birth Through Two Years, ND-10.
The Education of Children and Youth with Special Needs: What Do the Laws Say? ND-15.
Having a Daughter with a Disability: Is It Different for Girls? ND-14.
Learning Disabilities, ND-1.
The Least Restrictive Environment: Knowing One When You See It, ND-5.
Minority Issues Is Special Education, ND-9.
Parents' Guide to Vocational Education, ND-8.
Procedural Safeguards Ensuring That Handicapped Children Receive a Free Appropriate Public Education, ND-7.
Psychological Testing of Children with Disabilities, ND-2.
Respite Care: A Gift of Time, ND-12.
Social Skills, ND-6.

TRANSITION SUMMARY

Options After High School for Youth with Disabilities, TS-7.
Self Determination, TS-5.
Vocational Assessment, TS-6.

DISABILITY INFORMATION

Attention Deficit Disorder (Briefing Paper), FS-14.
Autism, FS-1.
Cerebral Palsy, FS-2.
Deafness, FS-3.
Down's Syndrome, FS-4.
Emotional Disturbance, FS-5.
Epilepsy, FS-6.
Learning Disabilities, FS-7.

Mental Retardation, FS-8.
Physical Disabilities & Special Health Problems, FS-9.
Severe and/or Multiple Handicaps, FS-10.
Speech and Language Impairments, FS-11.
Spina Bifida, FS-12.
Visual Impairments, FS-13.

MATERIALS FOR PARENTS

Life After School for Children with Disabilities: Answers to Questions Parents Ask About Employment and Financial Assistance, PA-5.
A Parent's Guide: Accessing the ERIC Resource Collection, PA-6.
A Parent's Guide: Accessing Special Education and Related Services: Communicating Through Letter Writing, PA-9.
A Parent's Guide: Planning a Move; Mapping Your Strategy, PA-8.
Parents' Guide to Accessing Parent Programs, Community Services, and Record Keeping, PA-3.
Parents' Guide to Accessing Programs for Infants, Toddlers, Preschoolers with Handicaps (Ages 0–5), PA-2.
A Parent's Guide to Doctors, Disabilities, and the Family, PA-7.

EASY-TO-READ

Help for Special Children (English), ER-1.
Help for Special Children (Spanish), ER-2.

LEGAL INFORMATION

Individualized Education Programs (IEP), LG-2.
Questions and Answers About How to Get Special Education Services for Your Child (Ages 3–21), LG-1.

NATIONAL LIBRARY SERVICES FOR THE BLIND AND PHYSICALLY HANDICAPPED, LIBRARY OF CONGRESS* *1-800-424-8567*
1291 Taylor St., N.W.
Washington, D.C. 20542

NATIONAL ORGANIZATION ON DISABILITY (NOD)* *1-800-248-ABLE*
910 16th St., N.W., Suite 600
Washington, D.C. 20006

*A federally supported clearinghouse related to disabilities.

NATIONAL REHABILITATION INFORMATION CENTER* 1-800-346-2742
8455 Colesville Road, Suite 935 *1-301-588-9284 Voice/TDD*
Silver Spring, MD 20910-3319

NEW ENGLAND ASSISTANCE DOG SERVICE, INC. (NEADS)* *1-508-835-3304 Voice/TDD*
P.O. Box 213
West Boylston, MA 01583

Purpose Hearing dogs are trained to alert deaf or hearing-impaired individuals to specific sounds in the environment. Sounds the dogs respond to include alarm clock, door bell, smoke alarm, telephone, baby crying, oven timer, car horn, and siren. *Service dogs* are trained to help people who use wheelchairs, canes, walkers, or crutches. These assistance dogs pick up anything dropped, pull wheelchairs, and carry items. *Specialty dogs* are trained to help people with two or more disabilities (an example might be a deaf person who uses a wheelchair).

Publications
New England Assistance Dog Service, a brochure.

PRESIDENT'S COMMITTEE ON EMPLOYMENT OF PEOPLE WITH DISABILITIES
1-202-376-6200 Voice
1-202-376-6205 TDD
Fax 1-202-376-6219
1331 F Street, N.W.
Washington, D.C. 20004-1107

Purpose The Americans with Disabilities Act of 1990 (ADA) makes it unlawful to discriminate in employment against a qualified individual with a disability. The ADA also outlaws discrimination against individuals with disabilities in state and local government services, public accommodations, transportation, and telecommunications. The President's Committee on Employment of People With Disabilities will answer questions from the disabled and from employers.

Publications
All public documents produced by the President's Committee on Employment of People with Disabilities are available on cassette tape, braille text, and large print.
Americans with Disability Act in Brief.
Americans with Disabilities Act in Brief: Focus on Employment.
Americans with Disabilities Act in Brief: Focus on Public Accommodations.
Americans with Disabilities Act in Brief: Focus on Telecommunications.
Americans with Disabilities Act in Brief: Focus on Transportation.
The Americans with Disabilities Act: Your Employment Rights as an Individual with a Disability.
Disabled Veterans: I Want You to Know About ADA.
Employers Are Asking About Accommodating Workers with Disabilities.

*A federally supported clearinghouse related to disabilities.

Fact Sheet on Aids in the Workplace and Its Impact on Health.
Fact Sheet on Employment Entrance Medical Examinations: Are They Beneficial and Legal?
Insurance and Other Corporate Policies Regarding Individuals with Disabilities.

OFFICE OF SPECIAL EDUCATION AND REHABILITATION SERVICES *1-202-732-1723*
U.S. Department of Education *1-202-732-1241 Voice/TDD*
Switzer Building, Room 3132
Washington, D.C. 20202-2524

Purpose Created by the Rehabilitation Act of 1973, the Clearinghouse responds to inquiries and researches and documents information operations serving the handicapped field on the national, state, and local levels. The Clearinghouse responds to inquiries on a wide range of topics. Information is especially strong in the areas of federal funding for programs serving individuals with disabilities, federal legislation affecting the handicapped community, and federal programs benefiting people with handicapping conditions. The Clearinghouse is knowledgeable about who has information and refers inquirers to appropriate sources.

Publications
The following publications are available free of charge from the Clearinghouse:

Information About the Office of Special Education and Rehabilitative Services, describes the program serving 4.4 million children and youth with disabilities and more than 930,000 adults with disabilities.

OSERS News in Print, a newsletter that focuses on federal activities affecting people with disabilities and new developments in the information field.

Pocket Guide to Federal Help for Individuals with Disabilities, a summary of benefits and services available to qualified individuals.

A Summary of Existing Legislation Affecting Persons with Disabilities, a history and description of all relevant laws through 1987.

WELL SPOUSE FOUNDATION
See under Homecare.

DIVERTICULOSIS
See Digestive Diseases.

DIZZINESS
See Vertigo.

DOMESTIC VIOLENCE
See Abuse.

DOWN'S SYNDROME

Occurs when a child is born with 47 chromosomes instead of 46. The syndrome is recognizable at birth. The baby has eyes that slope upward at the outer corners, the face and features are small, and the tongue is large and tends to stick out. Children with the syndrome are mentally retarded.

NATIONAL INSTITUTE OF CHILD HEALTH AND HUMAN DEVELOPMENT (NICHHD) — *1-301-496-5133*
Building 31, Room 2A32
Bethesda, MD 20892

Publications
Facts About Down's Syndrome.
Facts About Down's Syndrome for Women over 35, NIH Pub. No. 82-536.

DRUG ABUSE

Whether it is called drug "abuse," "habituation," "addiction," or "disorder," the reliance on mind altering chemicals is pervasive and tragic in our society. Since law enforcement is unable to control the illegal use of drugs, the best hope for keeping citizens from becoming enslaved by dependence on alcohol and drugs is education.

AMERICAN COUNCIL FOR DRUG EDUCATION — *1-301-294-0600*
204 Monroe St. — *Fax 1-301-294-0603*
Rockville, MD 20850 — *1-800-488-3784*

Purpose A national nonprofit membership organization with a Scientific Advisory Board, the Council provides facts and statistics on drugs and alcohol; has programs to prevent abuse in schools, families, and the workplace; and offers more than 70 pamphlets, monographs, films, and posters. It assists corporations and advertising agencies in developing cause-related marketing and community-based prevention programs. The Council also participates in national task forces and policy groups.

Publications
A Catalog of Membership Information & Materials.

CORPORATION AGAINST DRUG ABUSE (CADA) — *1-202-338-0654*
1010 Wisconsin Ave., N.W., Suite 250 — *Fax 1-202-338-0689*
Washington, D.C. 20007

Purpose CADA, a nonprofit organization of the private sector in metropolitan Washington, addresses the drug problem locally through workplace initiatives, community prevention strategies, and the establishment of regular and comprehensive reporting of data on substance abuse. CADA has created the Washington Employer Resource Consortium (WERC) to offer high-quality, low-cost employee assistance programs, testing packages, and managed health and mental health insurance to area employers. CADA's model youth prevention program is focused on 7th and 8th grade children in area school systems.

Publications

CADA Guide to a Drug-Free Workplace.

Drug-Free Workplace and Employee Assistance Services, answers questions about Employee Assistance Services, certified drug testing labs, and service hotlines.

Establishing a Drug-Free Workplace: A Legal Handbook Workplace.

DRUG ABUSE INFORMATION AND TREATMENT HOTLINE *1-800-662-HELP*

DRUG-FREE WORKPLACE HELPLINE *1-800-843-4971*

Purpose Trained information specialists are available from 9 A.M. to 8 P.M. EST, Monday through Friday, to offer advice and technical assistance on workplace programs.

Publications

Provides single copies of the following free:

Drugs in the Workplace: Research and Evaluation Data, Vol. II.

Drugs in the Workplace: Research and Evaluation Data, DHHS Pub. ADM 89-1612, 340 pages.

The Efficacy of Preemployment Drug Screening for Marijuana and Cocaine in Predicting Employment Outcome, by Craig Zwerling, James Ryan, and Endel John Orav, JAMA, Vol. 264, No. 20, 1990, pp. 2639–2643.

Urine Testing for Drugs of Abuse, edited by R. L. Hawks and C. N. Change, DHHS Pub. No. ADM 87-1481, 121 pages.

FAMILIES ANONYMOUS *1-818-989-7841*

P.O. Box 528
Van Nuys, CA 91408

Purpose This worldwide organization offers a 12-step, self-help program for families and friends of people with behavioral problems usually associated with drug abuse. The organization is similar in structure to Alcoholics Anonymous.

FEDERAL DRUG, ALCOHOL, AND CRIME CLEARINGHOUSE NETWORK *1-800-788-2800*
Number Linking Federal Services' Drug Abuse Information

Participating federal departments are

- Department of Health and Human Services
- Department of Education
- Department of Justice
- Department of Housing and Urban Development

The Clearinghouse Network is composed of the following:

- National Clearinghouse for Alcohol and Drug Information
- Drug Information and Treatment Referral Line
- Drug-Free Workplace Helpline
- Drugs & Crime Data Center and Clearinghouse
- Drug Information & Strategy Clearinghouse
- National AIDS Clearinghouse
- National Criminal Justice

Purpose With one call, you can now obtain the widest range of alcohol and other drug information currently available. Topics include addiction treatment information and referrals; prevention information, materials and curricula; alcohol and drug-related crime data and statistics; Drug-Free Workplace compliance information; research; database searches; posters; resources for parents and families; community action guides; fact sheets; impaired driving statistics; and many others.

JUST SAY NO INTERNATIONAL *1-415-939-6666*
1777 No. California Blvd., Suite 210 *Fax 1-415-933-8279*
Walnut Creek, CA 94596 *1-800-258-2766 (outside California)*

Publication

Formerly the Just Say No Foundation, "Just Say No" International provides direction and support to "Just Say No" clubs. The clubs are composed of groups of children, 7 to 14 years old, who are committed to leading drug-free lives and encourage their peers to do the same. The program includes education, recreation, social, community service, and outreach activities.

LIONS CLUBS INTERNATIONAL *1-708-571-5466*
300 22nd St. *Fax 1-708-571-8890*
Oak Brook, IL 60521-8842

Publication

Myth & Fact: Marijuana and You, a pamphlet refuting some of the myths about the drug.

NAR-ANON FAMILY GROUP HEADQUARTERS, INC. *1-213-547-5800*
WORLD SERVICE INTERNATIONAL
P.0. Box 2562
Palos Verdes, CA 90274

Although separate, Nar-Anon Family Groups is a companion program to Narcotics Anonymous.

NARCOTICS ANONYMOUS *1-818-780-3951*
P.O. Box 9999 *Fax 1-818-785-0923*
Van Nuys, CA 91409

Purpose Self-help organization of recovering drug addicts who meet regularly to help each other stay clean. There are no dues or fees for services. Meetings are available in 50 countries and throughout the United States. The only requirement for membership is the desire to stay clean.

NATIONAL CLEARINGHOUSE FOR ALCOHOL AND *1-301-468-2600*
DRUG INFORMATION (NCADI) *1-800-SAY-NO TO (drugs)*
Information Specialist
P.O. Box 2345
Rockville, MD 20852

Purpose The National Clearinghouse for Alcohol and Drug Information was established in 1987, when the National Clearinghouse for Alcohol Information and the National Clearinghouse for Drug Abuse Information were combined. The Clearinghouse gathers and disseminates current knowledge on alcohol and drug-related subjects. Services include searches on an in-house automated database and response to inquiries for statistics and other information. The Clearinghouse also develops resource materials and operates the Regional Alcohol and Drug Awareness Resource (RADAR) network, a nationwide linkage of drug information centers, and provides publications in bulk quantities to support local prevention and education programs. NCADI has developed an online database—IDA (Information on Drugs and Alcohol)—which has two major components, a prevention materials resource and a traditional bibliographic resource. The prevention materials component describes a variety of materials including, but not limited to, pamphlets, posters, videos, curricula, and booklets. The bibliographic component is made up of journal articles, books, reports, proceedings and conference papers, and other primary source materials. All materials in IDA are housed in the NCADI library. IDA is accessed through NCADI information specialists. The library is available and open to the public, Monday through Friday, 9:30 A.M.–4:30 P.M. The collection contains information on all aspects of alcohol and other drug abuse, including over 80 journals, newsletters, and major U.S. newspapers.

NATIONAL COCAINE HOTLINE *1-800-262-2463*
P.O. Box 100
Summit, NJ 07901

NATIONAL FAMILIES IN ACTION *1-404-934-6464*
2296 Henderson Mill Rd., Suite 300 *Fax 1-404-934-7137*
Atlanta, GA 30345

Purpose This nationwide, volunteer, grass-roots organization acts as a vehicle for ordinary citizens to organize to prevent drug abuse in their families and communities. Central to the group's activities is its National Drug Information Center, which houses 500,000 documents on drug abuse. The staff answers questions from concerned parents, friends, students, educators, the media, policymakers, and others. Information about drugs includes tobacco and alcohol provided by phone and mail and in person. Referrals to treatment centers are made.

Publications

American Prevention Movement, a 40-page booklet describes the success of grass-roots volunteers in the prevention movement since the 1970s.

Crack Update, a ten-panel brochure describing one of America's worst drugs.

Drug Abuse Update, a quarterly digest of accurate, reliable information about drug and alcohol abuse.

Drug Abuse Update for Kids, targets students in the middle and upper elementary grades. Four issues during the school year.

NATIONAL INSTITUTE ON DRUG ABUSE (NIDA) *1-800-662-HELP*
National Drug Information And Referral Line
5600 Fishers Lane
Rockville, MD 20857

NATIONAL INSTITUTES OF HEALTH (NIH) *1-301-496-2563*
Office of Clinical Center Communications
Building 10, Room 1C255
Bethesda, MD 20892

Publication

Drugs and the Brain, NIH Pub. No. 90-3172.

SEVENTH-DAY ADVENTIST COMMUNITY HEALTH SERVICES *1-516-627-2210*
P.O. Box 1029
Manhasset, NY 11030

Publication

Freedom from Addictions, the "Why's" of addiction with spiritual principles for freedom.

DRUG INFORMATION

See Medications.

DYSLEXIA

There is no universally accepted definition of dyslexia, but generally, it involves difficulty in learning to read despite conventional instruction, adequate intelligence, and sociocultural opportunity.

Signs that may signal dyslexia are

- Problems with reading, accuracy, speed, and comprehension
- Repeated spelling errors
- Reversal of letters when reading or writing
- Delayed spoken language
- Errors in letter naming
- Difficulty in learning and remembering printed words
- Cramped illegible handwriting
- Difficulty in telling left from right
- Lack of awareness of sounds in words
- Confusion about directions in space or time
- Difficulties in math

NATIONAL INSTITUTE OF CHILD HEALTH AND HUMAN DEVELOPMENT (NICHHD) *1-301-496-5133*
Building 31, Room 2A32
Bethesda, MD 20892

Publications

Developmental Dyslexia and Related Disorders, NIH Pub. No. 80-92 (reprinted January 1985).

Facts About Dyslexia.

ORTON DYSLEXIA SOCIETY *1-410-296-0232*
Chester Building, Suite 382 *1-800-ABCD-123 (outside Maryland)*
8600 LaSalle Road
Baltimore, MD 21204-6020

Purpose The society disseminates information about dyslexia. They send callers a packet of pamphlets and refer them to the Orton Dyslexia Society branch nearest them. Membership includes concerned parents, educators, physicians, researchers, diagnosticians, speech and language therapists, and others in the field, as well as the dyslexic individual.

Publications
Free pamphlets about dyslexia and the society.

DYSTONIA

Dystonia is a neurological disorder characterized by strong, involuntary muscle spasms that twist the body into unusual, painful, and disabling postures.

DYSTONIA MEDICAL RESEARCH FOUNDATION *1-213-852-1630*
8383 Wilshire Blvd., Suite 800
Beverly Hills, CA 90211

In Canada:
777 Hornby Street, Suite 1800 *1-604-661-4886*
Vancouver, B.C., Canada V6Z 2K3

Publication
Quarterly newsletter.

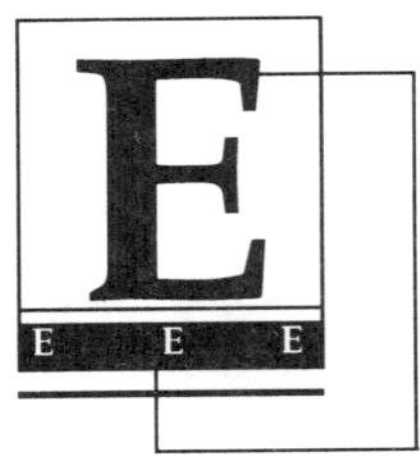

Ears

See also Deafness, Hearing Aids, *and* Tinnitus.

When the telephone rings a complex group of structures in your ear are set in motion, allowing you to hear the sound. The auricle, the outer ear, gathers the sound and passes it to your middle ear, an air-filled space between the eardrum and inner ear. When sound waves reach your eardrum, it shakes slightly, causing the bones of your middle ear to vibrate. This vibration moves the fluid in your inner ear, bending the tiny sensory hairs that covert sound to nerve impulses. These impulses are then carried to a "filing cabinet" in your brain, where stored memories enable you to recognize the sound as a telephone ringing.

AMERICAN ACADEMY OF OTOLARYNGOLOGY, HEAD AND NECK SURGERY (AAOHNS)
One Prince Street
Alexandria, VA 22314

1-703-836-4444
Fax 703-683-5100

Purpose The Academy is a nonprofit corporation whose membership represents approximately 98 percent of practicing otolaryngologists in the United States. Its function is to advance the science and art of medicine related to otolaryngology and represent the specialty in governmental and socioeconomic issues. Geographic lists of AAOHNS member physicians are available.

Publications

Send a stamped, self-addressed envelope for
Antihistamines, Decongestants and Cold Remedies.
Assistive Communication Devices Cochlear Implant.
Chain Saws and Your Safety.
Chew or Snuff Is Real Bad Stuff.
Cholesteatoma: A Serious Ear Condition.
Cold Sores, Fever Blisters, and Canker Sores.
A Discussion of Facial Nerve Problems.
Dizziness and Motion Sickness.
Doctor, What Causes the Noise in My Ears?
Earache and Otitis Media.
Ears, Altitude, and Airplane Travel.
Earwax.

Five-Minute Hearing Test.
Hayfever, Summer Colds and Allergies.
Head and Neck Cancer.
Is My Baby's Hearing Normal?
Noise, Ears and Hearing Protection.
Nosebleeds, Care & Prevention.
Pain and the TMJ.
Post Nasal Drip.
Sinus, Pain and Pressure.
Skull Base Surgery.
Smell & Taste Disorders.
Smokeless Tobacco: Is It Worth the Risk?
Smoking: The Hows and Whys of Quitting.
Snoring—Not Funny, Not Hopeless.
Sore Throats: Causes and Cures.
Swimmer's Ear, Itchy Ears, & Insects.
The Environment: Our Mutual Concern.
Tonsils & Adenoids.
Travel Tips for Hearing-Impaired People.
What Is an Otolaryngologist-Head and Neck Surgeon?
You and Your Stuffy Nose.
Your Medical Bills and Insurance Benefits.

AMERICAN SPEECH-LANGUAGE-HEARING ASSOCIATION *1-301-897-5700*
10801 Rockville Pike *1-800-638-8255*
Rockville, MD 20852

Purpose The Organization is a professional and scientific association of speech-language pathologists and audiologists, the professionals who treat communication disorders. Through toll-free consumer HELPLINE, the Association provides information about speech and hearing disorders and refers to speech-language pathologists and audiologists in requestor's area. The purposes of the Association are to encourage basic scientific study of the processes of individual human communication, with special reference to speech, hearing, and language; to promote investigation of disorders of human communication and to foster improvements of clinical procedures for such disorders; to stimulate exchange of information among persons and organizations thus engaged; and to disseminate information about communication disorders to the general public, physicians, and educators. Interested in the nature, processes, and disorders of speech, hearing, and language, including voice disorders, aphasia, cerebral palsy, cleft palate, delayed speech, laryngectomy, and stuttering; anatomy and physiology; auditory skills and training; psychoacoustics; audiometry; auditory feedback; hearing aids; phonetics; semantics; therapeutic techniques for speech and hearing disorders.

Publications

The following brochures are available:

American Speech-Language-Hearing Association Answers Questions About Adult Aphasia.

American Speech-Language-Hearing Association Answers Questions About Articulation Problems.

American Speech-Language-Hearing Association Answers Questions About Assistive Listening Devices.

American Speech-Language-Hearing Association Answers Questions About Child Language.

American Speech-Language-Hearing Association Answers Questions About Otitis Media.

American Speech-Language-Hearing Association Answers Questions About Otitis Medica, Hearing, and Language Development.

American Speech-Language-Hearing Association Answers Questions About Stuttering.

American Speech-Language-Hearing Association Answers Questions About Tinnitus.

American Speech-Language-Hearing Association Answers Questions About Voice Problems.

Communication Disorders And Aging.

Do Your Health Benefits Cover Audiology and Speech-Language Pathology Services?

Hearing Impairment and the Audiologist.

How Does Your Child Hear and Talk? Also available in Spanish.

Noise in Your Workplace.

Recognizing Communication Disorders.

Speech and Language Disorders and the Speech-Language Pathologist.

The Speech-Language Pathologist in the Schools.

EATING DISORDERS

Anorexia nervosa and its associated syndrome bulimia are extremely widespread problems. There are estimated to be more than a million victims in the United States. The conditions can be life-chronic and/or life threatening.

AMERICAN ANOREXIA/BULIMIA ASSOCIATION, INC. (AABA) *1-212-734-1114*
418 East 76th Street
New York, NY 10021

Purpose The Association provides information, referrals, and education on eating disorders; it also provides speakers and organizes conferences. Referrals are made to inpatient treatment centers, outpatient treatment centers, physicians, therapists, social workers, and self-help groups.

Publications
Quarterly newsletter.

ANOREXIA NERVOSA AND ASSOCIATED EATING DISORDERS (ANERD) *1-503-344-1144*
P.O. Box 5102
Eugene, OR 97405

Purpose The organization provides information and support to people with eating disorders and their families; also educates the general public about disordered eating and its prevention, holds workshops and training sessions for professionals and support groups, and refers to physicians specializing in eating disorders and to self-help groups.

Publications

Eating and Exercise Disorders, a booklet that provides more details than the brief brochure.

Eating Disorders, a brochure that lists symptoms and what to do about them.

NATIONAL ANOREXIC AID SOCIETY, INC. (NAAS) *1-614-436-1112*
1925 East Dublin-Graville Road
Columbus, OH 43229

Purpose The Society seeks to increase understanding and contribute toward the prevention of eating disorders. Provides information, education, professional training, and referral services for individuals with eating disorders, family, and friends to self-help organizations and professional treatment providers.

Publications

Center for the Treatment of Eating Disorders, a brochure.

Harding Hospital's Eating Disorders Program, a brochure.

National Anorexic Aid Society, a brochure.

NATIONAL ASSOCIATION OF ANOREXIA NERVOSA AND ASSOCIATED DISORDERS (NANAD) *1-708-831-3438*
P.O. Box 7
Highland Park, IL 60035

Purpose The organization was formed in 1976 to help assist individuals who suffer from anorexia nervosa/bulimia/compulsive eating and other eating disorders, as well as their families. NANAD has a large referral list of professionals who treat eating disorders as well as hundreds of support groups across the country and in nine foreign countries.

Publications

NANAD Working Together Newsletter.

Brief Descriptions of Some Therapies Used in Anorexia and Bulimia, information sheet including a bibliography.

Partial Listing of Physical Problems Brought About by Eating Disorders.

Some Suggestions About Finding a Therapist and Remaining in Therapy, information and a bibliography.

What Is Bulimia? information sheet including a bibliography.

NATIONAL INSTITUTE OF CHILD HEALTH AND HUMAN DEVELOPMENT (NICHHD) — *1-301-496-5133*
Building 31, Room 2A32
Bethesda, MD 20892

Publication

Facts About Anorexia Nervosa.

EHLERS-DANLOS SYNDROME (EDS)

See page 30.

EMERGENCIES

Everyone has experienced that breath-catching, heart-pounding, indecisive feeling known as "panic" when confronted with an emergency. The best ways to avoid the mental and physical short-circuiting that occurs during panic is to know what to do—how to cope with a situation that requires immediate action.

AMERICAN RED CROSS — *1-800-223-5000*
Eastern Operations Headquarters
P.O. Box 0549
Washington, D.C. 20073-0549

AMERICAN TRAUMA SOCIETY — *1-301-420-4189*, *1-800-556-7890*
8903 Presidential Parkway, Suite 512
Upper Marlboro, MD 20772-2656

Purpose Dedicated to the prevention of trauma and the improvement of trauma care as an education/awareness association.

Publications
Catalog listing educational materials for sale.

TRAUMAGRAM, newsletter incorporating society and prevention news.

MEDIC ALERT® FOUNDATION INTERNATIONAL
2323 Colorado
Turlock, CA 95380

1-209-668-3333
1-800-432-5378

Purpose This nonprofit organization provides personal medical information to protect and save lives. A bracelet or a necklace is engraved with medical conditions; a wallet card with your medical history is provided. Your medical history is stored on a computerized database and a 24-hour hotline is available to inform medical personnel of your medical history. Other services include Medic Alert® Response Service, a push button worn on the neck or wrist that provides two-way voice contact with emergency operators 24 hours a day, and International Implant Registry, which provides notification to patients and physicians of recalls and safety alerts for implanted medical devices such as pacemakers, orthopaedic devices, and breast implants. There is a small charge for the jewelry and updating the medical history, but the information about this important emergency service is free.

Publications
Medic Alert Applications.
Brochures including one of designer line Medic Alert® bracelets and necklaces.

EMPHYSEMA

See under National Jewish Center for Immunology and Respiratory Medicine.

ENDOMETRIOSIS

The tissue that lines the uterus, the endometrium, is shed as a menstrual period. In endometriosis, fragments of endometrium break loose and seed elsewhere. Each month these fragments of endometrium bleed like the lining of the uterus. But because the fragments are embedded in tissue, the blood cannot escape. As a result, blood blisters form that irritate and scar the surrounding tissue.

ENDOMETRIOSIS ASSOCIATION
8585 N. 76th Place
Milwaukee, WI 53223

1-800-992-ENDO

Purpose The Association is a self-help organization of women with endometriosis and others interested in exchanging information about the condition, offering mutual support and help to those affected by endometriosis, educating the public and medical community about the disease, and promoting research related to endometriosis. No referrals to physicians are made; however, networking opportunities among members are offered, which provides further opportunity for gathering information on local physicians.

Publications
Brochures are available in English, Spanish, French, Chinese, Japanese, and Dutch. The brochure provides information on endometriosis and the Endometriosis Association. There is also a brochure for teenagers.

NATIONAL INSTITUTE OF CHILD HEALTH AND HUMAN DEVELOPMENT (NICHHD) *1-301-496-5133*
Building 31, Room 2A32
Bethesda, MD 20892

Publication
Facts About Endometriosis, NIH Pub. No. 91-2413.

ENVIRONMENTAL HEALTH

The air we breathe and the substances we ingest or to which we expose our skin and eyes may affect our health. With increases in population, machines, chemicals, and airtight buildings, we need to inform ourselves about how to maintain a safe environment.

AMERICAN ACADEMY OF ENVIRONMENTAL MEDICINE (AAEM) *1-303-622-9755*
P.O. Box 16106 *Fax 1-303-622-4224*
Denver, CO 80216

Purpose This multispecialty medical society is involved with studying, treating, and preventing illnesses related to the environment. Readers may contact AAEM and request a list of member physicians in their region. They may also request a list of publications in the field of environmental medicine and referral to local patient support groups and national educational organizations involved with issues such as chemicals around the home or office.

AMERICAN INDUSTRIAL HYGIENE ASSOCIATION *1-216-873-2442*
345 White Pond Drive *Fax 1-216-873-1642*
Akron, OH 44320

Purpose The Association is a professional society for those practicing industrial hygiene in industry, government, labor, academic institutions, and independent organizations. Their goal is to keep workers, their families, and the community healthy and safe. It is the industrial hygienist's job to help ensure that federal, state, and local laws and regulations are followed in the work environment.

ARTS & CRAFTS MATERIALS INSTITUTE
715 Boylston Street
Boston, MA 12116
The Institute provides information of safety-approved and certified arts and crafts products.

CENTER FOR SAFETY IN THE ARTS, INC. *1-212-227-6220*
6 Beekman Street
New York, NY 10038

Purpose The Center—formerly the Center for Occupational Hazards—is a national clearinghouse for research and education on hazards in the visual arts, performing arts, educational facilities, and museums. The Center answers approximately 50 written and telephone inquiries daily on art hazards. Requests for information come from artists, craftspeople, theater technicians, performing artists, teachers, parents, students museum conservators, physicians, poison control centers, and government agencies. The Center researches the potential hazards of art materials and processes, writes and distributes publications on art hazards, and makes referrals to physicians with expertise in occupational medicine.

Publication

Is Your Art Hurting You? a sheet that explains the mission of the Center and the services offered. It also contains an order form for many publications ranging from 50 cents to $16 on specific materials and hazards.

CHEM TREC/CMA *1-800-262-8200 hotline*
Non-Emergency Service
2501 M Street, N.W.
Washington, D.C. 20037

Purpose Will answer questions about chemicals and has brochures available about specific chemicals when requested.

EDUCATIONAL COMMUNICATIONS, INC. *1-310-559-9160*
P.O. Box 351419
Los Angeles, CA 90035-9119

Purpose Educational Communications is a nonprofit organization funded by contributions, grants, and membership dues. The Ecology Center, one of its projects, serves as a regional environmental clearinghouse and conservation organization principally by evaluating environmental impact reports, distributing data, and providing testimony at governmental hearings. The environmental projects are concerned with toxics and chemicals and human health as well as wildlife, desert and forest management, and other environmental concerns. The Center is linked to the California Environmental Network database. The radio and television services research the public with the environmental message.

Publications
Fact sheets concerning services available and publications' list.
Compendium Newsletter.
Directory of Environmental Organizations.
More than 1,000 audio- and videocassettes.

HUMAN ECOLOGY ACTION LEAGUE, INC. *1-404-248-1898*
P.O. Box 49126
Atlanta, GA 30359

Purpose The Human Ecologist Action League collects and publishes information on human reactions to the environment. It is interested in adverse reactions to factors found in air, water, food, drugs, and habitat resulting in environmental illness. Its purpose is to serve those whose health has been adversely affected by environmental exposures, to provide information to those who are concerned about the health effects of chemicals, and to alert the general public about the potential dangers of chemicals.

Publications
Chemicals Can Affect Your Health, a brochure about the organization.
Listing of publications, a few offered free and the rest for a nominal fee.

NATIONAL CENTER FOR ENVIRONMENTAL HEALTH STRATEGIES *1-609-429-5358*
Mary Lamielle, Director
1100 Rural Ave.
Voorhees, NJ 08043

Purpose The Center provides a clearinghouse and technical, referral, support, and advocacy services for the public and those with environmentally and occupationally induced illnesses. NCEHS is involved in the elimination or minimization of toxic exposures in the home, workplace, school, and outdoor environment. Membership includes a newsletter, *The Delicate Balance.*

NATIONAL FOUNDATION FOR THE CHEMICALLY HYPERSENSITIVE 1-919-256-3591
P.O. Box 9
Wrightsville Beach, NC 28480

Purpose This nonprofit, volunteer organization is devoted to research, education, and dissemination of information about chemical hypersensitivity. It provides referrals to physicians and attorneys as well as advice and resource assistance for the chemically injured and their relatives.

Publications
Brochure on the National Foundation for the Chemically Hypersensitive.

NATIONAL INSTITUTE OF ENVIRONMENTAL HEALTH SCIENCES (NIEHS) 1-919-541-3345
P.O. Box 12233
Research Triangle Park, NC 27709

Publications

Human Health and the Environment—Some Research Needs, NIH Pub. No. 86-1277.

Issues and Challenges in Environmental Health, NIH Pub. No. 87-861.

National Institute of Environmental Health Sciences Research Programs, NIH Pub. No. 89-2225.

With Respect to Life: Protecting Human Health and the Environment Through Laboratory Animal Research.

NATIONAL INSTITUTES OF HEALTH (NIH) 1-301-496-2563
Office of Clinical Center Communications
Building 10, Room 1C255
Bethesda, MD 20892

Publication
Environment and Disease.

U.S. ENVIRONMENTAL PROTECTION AGENCY,
OFFICE OF AIR AND RADIATION; 1-703-308-8470
OFFICE OF ATMOSPHERIC AND INDOOR AIR PROGRAMS;
INDOOR AIR DIVISION.
Mail Code ANR-445W
401 M. Street, S.W.
Washington, D.C. 20460

Purpose The Indoor Air Division is responsible for a broad range of activities designated to support the development of national policies on indoor air pollution. The activities include data development, technical and policy analysis, information development and dissemination, training, and intra- and interagency issues pertaining to the impact of indoor air pollution and related topics on the public.

Publications

Current and Federal Indoor Air Quality Activities.

Director of State Indoor Air Contacts.

Fact Sheets

- *Environmental Tobacco Smoke (no. 5).*
- *Report to Congress Indoor Air Quality (no. 6).*
- *Residential Air Cleaners (no. 7).*
- *Sick Building Syndrome (no. 4).*
- *Use and Care of Home Humidifiers (no. 8).*
- *Ventilation and Air Quality in Offices (no. 3).*

The Inside Story—A guide to Indoor Air Quality.

Summary of Available Information on Residential Air Cleaning Devices.

EPIDERMOLYSIS BULLOSA

This is a group of inherited chronic noninflammatory skin diseases in which large bubbles and erosions result from slight injuries.

NATIONAL INSTITUTE OF ARTHRITIS AND MUSCULOSKELETAL AND SKIN DISEASES (NIAMSD) *1-301-496-8188*
Building 31, Room 4C05
Bethesda, MD 20892

Publication

Living With Epidermolysis Bullosa, NIH Pub. No. 84-663, a 31-page booklet.

EPILEPSY

Epilepsy results when brief periods of abnormal electrical impulses in the brain affect how brain cells function, which may change a person's awareness and movements. The result is a seizure or convulsion. In about half of all cases, no cause is ever discovered. Depending on how well the therapy controls the seizures, a person can work full time and participate in most sports.

EPILEPSY FOUNDATION OF AMERICA
4351 Garden City Dr., Suite 406
Landover, MD 20785

1-301-459-3700
1-800-EFA-1000,
Information and referral only

Purpose The Epilepsy Foundation of America is the national, voluntary health organization dedicated to the prevention and cure of seizure disorders, the alleviation of their effects, and the promotion of independence and an optimal quality of life for people who have these disorders. The Foundation seeks to accomplish this mission through support of research, education, advocacy, and service. The Foundation provides education, advocacy, employment-related programs, publications, and the National Epilepsy Library and supports research. It refers to physicians and local EFA affiliates and other public and private social service agencies.

Publications
Catalog of publications available on the subject.
Epilepsy Foundation of America.
National Epilepsy Library.

NATIONAL INSTITUTE OF NEUROLOGICAL DISORDERS AND STROKE (NINDS)
Building 31, Room 8A06
Bethesda, MD 20892

1-301-496-5751

Publication
Epilepsy, NIH Pub. No. 81-0156.

NATIONAL INSTITUTES OF HEALTH (NIH)
Office of Clinical Center Communications
Building 10, Room 1C255
Bethesda, MD 20892

1-301-496-2563

Publications
Epilepsy, NIH Pub. No. 82-2369.
Understanding Seizure Disorders, a videotape that can be borrowed.

ESTROGEN
See under Aging.

EYES
See also under Blindness, Aging *and* Diabetes

Your eyes give you more information than any of your other sense organs, and thus your brain awards it more space than the other four main senses. Your eyes are complex and delicate. They are also the "windows" of the body and the mind.

AMERICAN OPTOMETRIC ASSOCIATION *1-314-991-4100*
243 N. Lindbergh Blvd. *Fax 1-314-991-4101*
St. Louis, MO 63121

Publications

Send a stamped, self-addressed, business-size envelope for

Are Your Eyes Safe from UV Radiation? tells you the importance of protecting your eyes from ultraviolet radiation.

Do Vision Problems Cause Adult Reading Problems? describes vision skills needed for good reading performance.

Family Guide to Vision Care, discusses the myth of 20/20 vision and how to select eye glasses.

Your Baby's Eyes, pamphlet about helping your baby develop hand-eye coordination and depth perception.

Your Preschool Child's Eyes, describes how you can handle your child's first eye examination visit and how to assess your child's vision.

Your School-Age Child's Eyes, pamphlet that helps parents be alert for symptoms that may indicate a child has a vision problem affecting school work.

VDT User's Guide to Better Vision, gives hints about working more comfortably and safely with a computer screen.

LIONS CLUBS INTERNATIONAL *708-571-5466*
300 22nd St. *Fax 708-571-8890*
Oak Brook, IL 60521-8842

Purpose Founded in 1917 and with 1.4 million volunteers worldwide, the Lions Clubs make possible 20,000 corneal transplants each year and, among other charitable endeavors, promote skills for adolescents and grade school children.

NATIONAL EYE INSTITUTE *1-301-496-5248*
Building 31, Room 6A32
Bethesda, MD 20892

Publications

Age-Related Macular Degeneration, NIH Pub. No. 89-2294, describes the eye disease that affects the macula, a small portion of the light-sensing retina. It is present to at least a mild degree in millions of older Americans. It is a leading cause of visual loss in this country.

Cataracts, NIH Pub. No. 89-201, a brochure that describes current treatments for cataract, a cloudy or opaque area in the lens of the eye.

Diabetic Retinopathy, NIH Pub. No. 90-2171, 10 million Americans have diabetes and should know the effects that condition may have on their eyes and the ways to prevent or lessen damage.

Glaucoma, NIH Pub. No. 89-651, 2 million Americans suffer from this eye disease that involves fluid pressure inside the eye and that if left untreated, can lead to blindness.

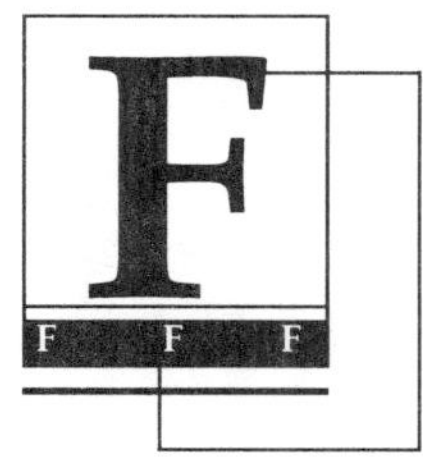

Facial Nerve Problems

Neuralgia is a painful condition in a nerve due to some unknown irritation or inflammation. *Trigeminal neuralgia* or *Tic douloureux* is the most common form of neuralgia and is characterized by repeated attacks of excruciating pain in one side of the face, usually involving the lips and nose most severely, sometimes also the gums and tongue.

American Academy of Otolaryngology, Head and Neck Surgery (AAOHNS) — *703-836-4444*, *Fax 703-683-5100*
One Prince Street
Alexandria, VA 22314

Publication
Send a stamped, self-addressed envelope for
A Discussion of Facial Nerve Problems

Familial Multiple Endocrine Neoplasia Type 1

This condition involves tumors of the parathyroid gland in the neck, the pancreas, and the pituitary.

National Institute of Diabetes and Digestive and Kidney Diseases (NIDDKD) — *1-301-499-3583*
Building 31, Room 9A04
Bethesda, MD 20892

Publication
Familial Multiple Endocrine Neoplasia Type 1, NIH Pub. No. 89-3048.

FDA (Food and Drug Administration)

HFE88 — *1-301-443-3170*
5600 Fishers Lane
Rockville, MD 20857

Publication

Getting Information from FDA, (FDA No. 91-1167), reprint of FDA Consumer article.

FEET

Your foot contains 26 bones and 33 junctures joined together by over 100 ligaments. Nineteen muscles provide power and control of the foot. The bones are arranged in two arches—a lengthwise arch and a crosswise arch. Your feet support the whole weight of your body and act as levers as you move forward in walking or running.

AMERICAN PODIATRIC MEDICAL ASSOCIATION — *1-301-571-9200*
9312 Old Georgetown Road — *1-800-FOOTCARE*
Bethesda, MD 20814-1621 — *Fax 1-301-530-2752*

Purpose The Association provides consumers with pamphlets on various subjects pertaining to foot health. It is not a referral line. A leaflet accompanies pamphlets giving the consumers information about how to find telephone information about doctors of podiatric medicine.

Publications

Podiatric Medicine: The Profession, The Physician, the Practice.
Your Podiatrist Talks About Aging.
Your Podiatrist Talks About Arthritis.
Your Podiatrist Talks About Athlete's Foot.
Your Podiatrist Talks About Children's Feet.
Your Podiatrist Talks About Diabetes.
Your Podiatrist Talks About Foot and Ankle Injuries.
Your Podiatrist Talks About Foot Health.
Your Podiatrist Talks About Foot Orthoses.
Your Podiatrist Talks About Foot Surgery.
Your Podiatrist Talks About Heel Pain.
Your Podiatrist Talks About High Blood Pressure.
Your Podiatrist Talks About Medicare.
Your Podiatrist Talks About Nail Problems.
Your Podiatrist Talks About On-the-Job Foot Health.
Your Podiatrist Talks About Walking.
Your Podiatrist Talks About Warts.
Your Podiatrist Talks About Women's Feet.

MYCELEX® OTC
444 N. Michigan Avenue, Suite 1600
Chicago, IL 60611

Publication

Put Your Best Foot Forward: Fending Off Fungal Skin Infections. The tips contained in this booklet were developed with the expert advice of Rodney S. W. Basler, M.D., chairman, Task Force on Sports Medicine for the American Academy of Dermatology and Miles' Consumer Health Care Division.

NATIONAL INSTITUTES OF HEALTH (NIH) *1-301-496-2563*
Office of Clinical Center Communications
Building 10, Room 1C255
Bethesda, MD 20892

Publication

Your Problem Feet: Care and Management, a videotape that can be borrowed.

FEVER BLISTERS AND CANKER SORES

Cold sores or "fever blisters" are produced by the herpes simplex virus. Canker sores are little blisters on membranes of the mouth and cheeks which break and leave open sores. They are believed to be caused by a bacteria.

NATIONAL INSTITUTE ON DEAFNESS AND OTHER COMMUNICATION DISORDERS (NIDOCD) *1-301-496-7243*
Building 31, Room 1B62
Bethesda, MD 20892

Publication

Fever Blisters and Canker Sores, NIH Pub. No. 87-247.

FIBROMYALGIA (FIBROSITIS, FMS)

A widespread musculoskeletal pain and fatigue disorder for which the cause is still unknown. "Fibromyalgia" means pain in the muscles, ligament, and tendons—the fibrous tissues in the body. FMS used to be called the fibrositis syndrome, implying there was inflammation in the muscles, but that has not been borne out by research. Most patients with FMS say they ache all over. Sometimes the muscles twitch, and at other times they burn. More women than men are afflicted with FMS, but it shows up in people of all ages.

FIBROMYALGIA NETWORK 1-800-631-1950
5700 Stockdale Hwy., Suite 100
Bakersfield, CA 93309

Purpose The Network provides information on the fibromyalgia syndrome, the chronic fatigue syndrome, and related disorders. Self-help group/patient contacts and health care referrals are provided for a stamped, self-addressed envelope.

Publication
FMS: A Patient Guide Brochure.

FITNESS
See under Physical Fitness.

FLU
See also under Aging.

Influenza is caused by a virus that spreads from one person to another in the spray from coughs and sneezes. The virus enters the upper part of the respiratory tract through the nose or mouth, and it may also invade the rest of the tract, including the lungs. Symptoms appear after an incubation period of one or two days. Influenza is usually an epidemic disease occurring in winter or early spring and affecting many people within a community.

NATIONAL INSTITUTE OF ALLERGY AND INFECTIOUS DISEASES (NIAID) 1-301-496-5717
Building 31, Room 7A32
Bethesda, MD 20892

Publication
Flu, NIH Pub. No. 87-187.

FOOD
See Nutrition and Diet.

FRAGILE X

An estimated 30 to 50 percent of males institutionalized because of mental retardation are said to have X-linked mutant genes that cause their condition. Some of these males have an X chromosome with a pinch near the end of the long arm with a small knob separated from the main portion of the chromosome by a thin stalk.

NATIONAL FRAGILE X FOUNDATION
1441 York St., Suite 250
Denver, CO 80206

1-303-333-6155
1-800-688-8765
Fax 1-303-333-4369

Purpose The Foundation promotes the education and research regarding fragile X syndrome, a genetic disorder which is the leading cause of inherited mental retardation. Offers a nationwide information and referral services. There are 42 resource centers in the United States and Canada that are affiliated with the Foundation. Referrals are made to physicians, genetic counselors, educators, and special education therapists are made on an individual basis.

Publications

The "family packet" has been designed for families diagnosed with fragile X or families who suspect they may have fragile X.

The "professional packet" is aimed at professionals who work with fragile X individuals and their families. Specific information pertaining to speech and language and occupational therapies is included in the packets.

FRIEDREICH'S ATAXIA

In this condition, unsteady walking begins between the ages of 5 and 15 years followed by arm incoordination and other symptoms such as a twisted spinal column and heart problems.

NATIONAL INSTITUTE OF NEUROLOGICAL DISORDERS AND STROKE (NINDS)
Building 31, Room 8A06
Bethesda, MD 20892

1-301-496-5751

Publication

Friedreich's Ataxia, NIH Pub. No. 82-87.

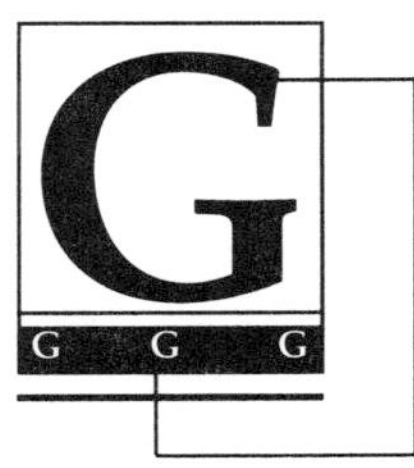

GALLBLADDER

See also Digestive Problems.

The gallbladder is a saclike organ underlying the liver in which bile, which helps to process fats, is stored, concentrated and delivered to the digestive tract as needed.

NATIONAL INSTITUTE OF DIABETES AND DIGESTIVE AND KIDNEY DISEASES (NIDDKD) *1-301-499-3583*
Building 31, Room 9A04
Bethesda, MD 20892

Publication

Gallstones, NIH Pub. No. 87-2897.

GAMBLING

Gambling, according to Gamblers Anonymous, is an illness. A compulsive gambler is described as a person whose gambling has caused growing and continuing problems in any department of his or her life. Some danger signals are

- An inability to stop gambling whether winning or losing and constant vows to abstain
- Impatience with loved ones
- Fantasies of "this week's win" to overcome "last week's loss" and dreams of "bigger wins"
- The neglect of responsibility to concentrate on gambling activities
- Perpetual statement, "Don't worry about it!"
- Lack of interest in social situations
- Belief that life without gambling is impossible

COUNCIL ON COMPULSIVE GAMBLING *1-609-599-3299*
1315 W. State Street *1-800-GAMBLER*
Trenton, NJ 08618

Purpose The Council provides nationwide, 24-hour hotline with referrals to treatment centers and Gamblers Anonymous meetings throughout the country.

GAMBLERS ANONYMOUS *1-213-386-8789*
Box 17173
Los Angeles, CA 90017

Purpose Gamblers Anonymous is a fellowship of thousands of men and women who have joined together to do something about their own gambling problem and to help other compulsive gamblers do the same.

Publications

Gamblers Anonymous, a history of the fellowship and its recovery and unity programs.
Gamblers Anonymous: Questions and Answers About the Problem of Compulsive Gambling and the G.A. Recovery Program.
Gambling Problem? There Is Help! A brochure about Gamblers Anonymous.
Young Gamblers In Recovery.

GAS (INTESTINAL)

A normal bowel always contains some gas but excessive amounts released by belching or passing wind, may result from indiscretions of diet or some disorder of the digestive system.

NATIONAL INSTITUTE OF DIABETES AND DIGESTIVE AND KIDNEY DISEASES (NIDDKD) *1-301-499-3583*
Building 31, Room 9A04
Bethesda, MD 20892

Publication

Gas in the Digestive Tract, NIH Pub. No. 90-883.

GASTROINTESTINAL PROBLEMS

See Digestive Diseases.

GENETIC COUNSELING

One of the fastest-developing areas of medical science concerns genetics and the understanding of how inherited diseases are carried from generation to generation.

Interventions are now being developed so that a "gene," the carrier of hereditary information, can be corrected if it is defective. In the meantime, there are counseling services to help couples who are concerned about the possibility of having a child with an inherited disease or defect.

ALLIANCE OF GENETIC SUPPORT GROUPS — *1-202-331-0942*
1001 22nd Street, N.W., Suite 800 — *1-800-336-GENE*
Washington, D.C. 20037 — *Fax 1-202-293-0479*

Purpose To serve a national coalition of voluntary genetic support groups, to provide a system of interchange between genetic professionals and consumers, and to advocate for and educate about people with genetic conditions. Serves as a clearinghouse for referral to genetic support groups and to genetic counselors.

Publications
Brochure about the Alliance.
Guide to National Voluntary Genetic Organizations.
Health Insurance Resource Guide.

EMANUEL HOSPITAL AND HEALTH CENTER — *1-503-280-4726*
2801 N. Gantenbein — *1-503-280-3033 Hotline*
Portland, OR 97227

Purpose Teratogen information referral line. (Teratogenesis involves the production of a malformed fetus.) Provides counseling and testing and prenatal diagnosis.

HEALTH AND HUMAN SERVICES, DEPARTMENT OF; — *1-301-496-5844*
PUBLIC HEALTH SERVICE; NATIONAL INSTITUTES OF HEALTH;
NATIONAL HEART, LUNG, AND BLOOD INSTITUTE;
LABORATORY OF MOLECULAR HEMATOLOGY
Building 10, Room 7D-18
Bethesda, MD 20892

Purpose The agency answers inquiries, provides advisory services and information on research in progress, conducts seminars and workshops, analyzes data on the following genetic conditions and therapies: adenosine diaminase (ADA), ADA deficiency, severe combined immunodeficiency (SCID), Cooley's anemia, thalassemia, molecular biology, molecular genetics, deoxyribonucleic acid (DNA), ribonucleic acid (RNA), globin, gene expression, protein biosynthesis, recombinant DNA technology, molecular cloning, gene therapy, genetic engineering, gene transfer, retroviruses, retroviral-mediated gene transfer, transcription factors, and DNA-protein interactions. Distributes publications; makes referrals to other sources of information. Services are free and available to anyone.

Publications
Books, technical reports, journal articles, state-of-the-art reviews, critical reviews, research summaries,bibliographies, and reprints.

NATIONAL INSTITUTES OF HEALTH (NIH) *1-301-496-2563*
Office of Clinical Center Communications
Building 10, Room 1C255
Bethesda, MD 20892

Publications
Control and Therapy of Genetic Diseases, a videotape that can be borrowed free of charge.
The Genetics of Cancer, NIH Pub. No. 90-3056.

GENETICS
See also Cleft Lip and Palate Foundation, Cooley's Anemia Foundation, Fragile X Foundation, Gluten Intolerance Association, Hemochromatosis Foundation, Joseph's Disease, Lowe's Syndrome, Marfan's Syndrome, Neurofibromatosis, Spina Bifida/Torsion Dystonia, Tay-Sach and Allied Diseases, Tuberous Sclerosis, Turner's Syndrome.

GERONTOLOGY
See Aging.

GINGIVITIS
See Gum Disease.

GLAUCOMA
Glaucoma is an eye disease that involves fluid pressure inside the eye and may lead to blindness if untreated.

FOUNDATION FOR GLAUCOMA RESEARCH (FGR) *1-415-986-3162*
490 Post Street, Suite 830
San Francisco, CA 94102

Purpose The Foundation seeks to protect the sight of individuals with glaucoma through research and education. Provides patient education information and referrals to physicians who are members of the American Glaucoma Society. The FGR also has information on support groups, provides seed money for research, and conducts basic and clinical research.

Publications

Fact sheets on various aspects of glaucoma.

Informational brochures, including *Glaucoma Research Eye Donor Network* brochure.

Newsletter, reporting latest information for patients, health care professionals, and family members of glaucoma patients.

Understanding and Living with Glaucoma, a patient education and reference guide.

INTERNATIONAL ASSOCIATION OF LIONS CLUBS
300 22nd St.
Oak Brook, IL 60570-0001

Publication

Glaucoma.

GLUTEN INTOLERANCE

See also Diet *and* Nutrition.

Celiac sprue, also known as gluten-sensitive enteropathy, non-tropical spruce, and celiac disease, is one of many digestive diseases. In the United States, it is thought to affect 1 person in every 2,500. Caucasians of Northern European ancestry are more often affected. In this inherited disorder, the lining of the small intestine is affected. Damage to the lining occurs when certain proteins, containing gliadin, are eaten. Gliadin-containing proteins are found in wheat, rye, barley, and oats. When damage to the lining of the small intestine occurs, many nutrients in food cannot be digested and absorbed normally. A wide range of symptoms may occur, including diarrhea, bloating, weight loss, anemia, and chronic fatigue.

GLUTEN INTOLERANCE GROUP OF NORTH AMERICA (GIG) *1-206-325-6980*
P.O. Box 23053
Seattle, WA 98102-0353

Purpose GIG offers assistance to those with celiac sprue and/or dermatitis herpetiformis, their families, and health care professionals through publications, seminars, videotapes, and telephone counseling, and referral. Refers to physicians and provides local contact people, product and drug information, and research assistance.

Publications

Brochure describing celiac sprue, symptoms, diagnosis, and treatment.

Publication lists of books and information packets for sale.

GOUT

See under Arthritis.

GROWTH

Most short children do not have a serious growth problem. Many grow at a normal rate and reach an adult height that is about the same as their parents'. A child's rate of growth is an important clue to the presence or absence of a growth problem. There are many conditions and diseases that can cause poor growth. Signals that you may need an expert professional examination for your child are if

- He or she is the shortest in the class.
- He or she is still wearing last year's clothes.
- She or he is unable to keep up with the other kids their age at play.
- He or she is growing less than 2 inches per year.

HUMAN GROWTH FOUNDATION *1-703-883-1772*
7777 Leesburg Pike, Suite 202S *1-800-451-6434*
Falls Church, VA 22043

Purpose The Foundation seeks to create public awareness about presence and treatability of growth disorders, particularly in children; support nationwide network of local chapters; and fund research in the area of growth disorders. It also makes referrals to specialists in your locale.

Publications

Achondroplasia, a child may fail to grow because of a primary bone disorder, a condition that affects 1 child in every 40,000 births.

Intrauterine Growth Retardation, points out that the most common cause of small size at birth is prematurity but that some full-term babies are markedly short and underweight at birth. Discusses the possible reasons.

Growth Hormone Deficiency, a booklet explaining the various causes of growth problems.

Patterns of Growth, describes general growth rates of children as well as an overview of several different growth disorders.

Short and OK: A Guide for Parents of Short Children, explores the psychosocial aspects of normal and abnormal short stature in children.

Turner Syndrome, describes the genetic disorder that results from an abnormality of a chromosome.

GUILLAIN-BARRE SYNDROME (GBS)

Guillain-Barre syndrome, also called idiopathic polyneuritis and Landry's ascending paralysis, is an inflammatory disorder of the peripheral nerves, those outside the brain and spinal cord. It involves a rapid onset of weakness and often paralysis of the legs, arms, breathing muscles, and face. Abnormal sensations may accompany the weakness. GBS can develop in any person at any age.

GUILLAIN-BARRE SYNDROME FOUNDATION INTERNATIONAL *1-215-667-0131*
P.O. Box 262
Wynnewood, PA 19096

Purpose Founded in 1981 by Robert and Estelle Benson to help others deal with a frightening and potentially catastrophic disorder from which recovery is uncertain, the Foundation has more than 130 chapters nationally and internationally. Its goals are to help GBS patients and their families. Visits are made to patients by recovered GBS individuals. The Foundation provides research funding and will refer to physicians and self-help groups in requestor's area.

Publications

The Communicator, a newsletter.

Guillain-Barre Syndrome, a brochure about the condition and the organization.

Guillain-Barre Syndrome, a 44-page booklet that gives an overview for the layperson of the syndrome, its diagnosis, and treatment.

GUM DISEASE

Inflamed and swollen gums (gingivitis) are usually caused by plaque, a sticky deposit of mucus, food particles, and bacteria that forms around the bottom of the teeth. It may also be caused by a vitamin deficiency, by certain medications, and by some glandular disorders and blood diseases. Gingivitis is very common in adults, pregnant women, and diabetics. Gum disease is one of the most common causes of tooth loss.

AMERICAN ACADEMY OF PERIODONTOLOGY *1-312-787-5518*
737 North Michigan Ave., Suite 800
Chicago, IL 60611-2690

Purpose The American Academy of Periodontology is a 6,200-member association of dental professionals specializing in the prevention, diagnosis, and treatment of diseases affecting the gums and supporting structures of the teeth. The Academy serves as an educational resource for periodontists and general dentists and is committed to increasing the public's awareness of periodontal disease and how it can be prevented and treated. Will refer to periodontists in your locale.

Publications

To obtain single copies of any brochure, send a stamped, self-addressed, business-sized envelope to the above address, Attention Dept. PH. Indicate on the outer envelope which brochure(s) you are requesting.

Dental Implants: Are They Right For You? a brochure designed for the patient considering dental implants, that illustrates different types of dental implants and explains how implants are used to correct a variety of dental problems.

Gum Disease: Be Tested to See If You Have It, a pamphlet that stresses early detection and treatment, describes how gum disease progresses, and explains what is included in a thorough periodontal exam.

Gum Disease: What You Need to Know, a brochure that serves as a guide to the causes, treatment, and prevention of periodontal disease. Also available in Spanish.

How to Brush and Floss, a brochure that provides easy-to-follow instructions on brushing and flossing and stresses the importance of regular dental visits.

Keeping Your Gums Healthy, a brochure designed for the patient who has completed the active phase of periodontal treatment. It answers some of the most frequently asked questions about maintenance therapy.

Periodontal Surgery: What Can I Expect? a brochure that explains when periodontal surgery may be needed, when to return to the periodontist, and what methods can be used to prevent the recurrence of the disease.

GYNECOLOGY

See Endometriosis, Pregnancy, *and* Women's Health.

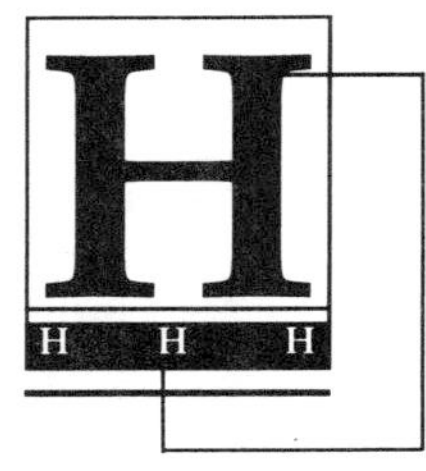

HANDICAPPED

See Disabilities.

HEADACHE

Everyone has had a headache sometime or other. A report in *The Journal of the American Medical Association*, January 1, 1992, estimated that 8.7 million females and 2.6 million males suffer from migraine headache with moderate to severe disability. Of these, 3.4 million females and 1.1 million males experience one or more attacks per month. There are many other causes of headache, and if the attack is severe or persistent, immediate medical evaluation is indicated.

AMERICAN ACADEMY OF PEDIATRICS
Department C, P.O. Box 927
Elk Grove Village, IL 60009-0927

Publication
Send a stamped, self-addressed, business-size envelope for *Important Information for Teens Who Get Headaches.*

MONTEFIORE MEDICAL CENTER *1-212-920-4636*
Headache Unit Neurology Department
111 East 210th St.
Bronx, NY 10467

Purpose The Center seeks to diagnose and treat headache disorders and conduct research into the cause and control of headaches.

Publications
Brochure about the Headache Unit.

NATIONAL HEADACHE FOUNDATION (NHF) *1-312-878-7715*
5252 North Western Ave. *1-800-843-2256*
Chicago, IL 60625

Purpose The Foundation is a nonprofit organization with three major goals:

1. To serve as an information source to headache sufferers, their families, and the physicians who treat them
2. To promote research into potential headache causes and treatments
3. To educate the public to the fact that headaches are serious disorders and the sufferers need understanding and continuity of care

Publications

Send a stamped (two first class), self-addressed, business-size envelope for a free copy of the newsletter and a list of NHF physician members. Briefly mention your headache type and symptoms if undiagnosed. The organization also has a number of publications for sale.

NATIONAL INSTITUTE OF NEUROLOGICAL DISORDERS AND STROKE (NINDS) *1-301-496-5751*
Building 31, Room 8A06
Bethesda, MD 20892

Publication

Headache, NIH Pub. No. 84-158.

HEAD INJURIES

A head injury is defined as an insult to the brain caused by an external physical force that may or may not produce a diminished or altered state of consciousness. A head injury may result in disturbance of behavior or emotional functioning. These impairments may be either temporary or permanent and may cause partial or total functional disability or psychological maladjustment. About half a million persons are hospitalized each year with a head injury, about 50 percent of them due to motor vehicle accidents. Males outnumber females 3 to 1.

NATIONAL HEAD INJURY FOUNDATION, INC. *1-800-444-6443*
1776 Massachusetts Ave., N.W., Suite 100
Washington, D.C. 20036

Purpose The Foundation seeks to improve the quality of life of survivors of head injury and their families and to promote the prevention of head injury. The family helpline listed is a direct link to the Information and Resources Department, whose staff answer questions about head injury and its consequences, provide detailed information about specific aspects of brain injury through access to the Foundation's library, and provide referrals to providers of rehabilitation services nationwide.

Publication
Catalog of publications.

NATIONAL INSTITUTE OF NEUROLOGICAL DISORDERS AND STROKE (NINDS) — *1-301-496-5751*
Building 31, Room 8A06
Bethesda, MD 20892

Publication
Head Injury, NIH Pub. No. 84-2478.

HEALTH CARE COSTS

There are approximately 1,500 health insurance companies in the United States, covering 189 million Americans. The United States General Accounting Office estimates that $67 billion could be saved each year if the United States adopted a single payer system such as Canada's. On the other hand, even Canadian citizens admit their system is not perfect.

AMERICAN ACADEMY OF OTOLARYNGOLOGY HEAD AND NECK SURGERY (AAOHNS) — *703-836-4444*, *Fax 703-683-5100*
One Prince Street
Alexandria, VA 22314

Publication
Send a stamped, self-addressed envelope for
Your Medical Bills and Insurance Benefits.

AMERICAN COUNCIL OF LIFE INSURANCE (ACLI) — *1-202-624-2000*, *1-800-942-4242 Helpline*
1001 Pennsylvania Ave., N.W.
Washington, D.C. 20004

Purpose The mission of the ACLI is to provide a unified association to advance the interest of the life insurance industry; to assure effective government relations at both federal and state levels; and to engage in other activities for the education, information, and assistance of its members and the public. It publishes and provides life insurance information to consumers and sponsors consumer helpline listed.

Publication
Accelerated Death Benefit Products, a 12-page booklet concerning accelerated benefits, also known as living benefits, which are life insurance policy proceeds paid to the policyholder *before* he or she dies. The benefits may be provided for in

the policies themselves, but more often they are specified in attachments or riders that are added to new or existing policies.

Consumers Guide to Life Insurance, a 20-page booklet about life insurance, and types of policies; includes a form for assessing your financial worth and a glossary.

HEALTH INSURANCE ASSOCIATION OF AMERICA *1-202-223-7780*
P.O. Box 41455 *1-800-942-4242*
Washington, D.C. 20018

Purpose The Association serves as the forum for developing policy that reflects broad consensus and support within the industry. It also represents the industry in work with legislators and regulators; conducts research and publishes technical literature and policy analyses on developments and trends; serves the consumer through publication of its consumer guides to health, disability, Medigap, and long-term care insurance; and sponsors consumer helpline to answer questions on related topics.

Publications

Consumers Guide to Disability Insurance, a 12-page booklet defining disability insurance and what steps you should take if you need it.

Consumer's Guide to Health Insurance, a 16-page booklet that offers information and advice on private health insurance and suggests ways to use your health insurance dollar wisely. It is aimed particularly at helping those with little or no group protection.

Consumers Guide to Long-Term Care Insurance, a 24-page booklet that provides a list of companies selling long-term care insurance; tells you what you should know before you buy and what policies do and do not cover. Also includes a checklist and a glossary.

Consumers Guide to Medicare Supplemental Insurance (Medigap), a 20-page booklet about what is covered and what is not covered by Medicare and what coverage is available to supplement it. Includes a glossary.

Health Insurance: A Guide for Small Business Owners, a kit including a checklist for comparing plans and hints on holding down costs.

PEOPLE'S MEDICAL SOCIETY (PMS) *1-215-770-1670 Information*
462 Walnut Street (lower level) *1-800-624-8773 Orders only*
Allentown, PA 18102

Purpose The People's Medical Society, founded in 1983, is a membership organization encouraging active involvement by patients in their own medical care. It advocates a ten-point code of practice for practitioners, which emphasizes fairness in fees and open communication with patients. The PMS offers advice to medical consumers about reducing costs and improving the quality and safety of care through its newsletter and other publications. The Society opposes unnecessary therapies and procedures, advocates access to medical records, and encourages patients to be fully informed about their conditions and the treatments they undergo. The PMS is a not-for-profit organization that provides information and referrals to self-help groups.

Publication
A list of publications for sale.

HEALTH INFORMATION

Obtaining information about a personal medical problem is the first step in being an aware and effective medical consumer.

AMERICAN INDIAN HEALTH CARE ASSOCIATION (AIHCA) *1-612-293-0233*
245 East Sixth Street, Suite 499
St. Paul, MN 55101

Purpose The Association serves as a national voice, an information clearinghouse, a research agent, and a source of planning technical assistance and training for Indian health programs across the United States. The AIHCA seeks to develop, promote, and support high-quality and culturally sensitive health services for American Indian people. It provides training for American Indian health care providers, offers technical assistance, and conducts research concerning effective health promotion strategies.

Publications
AIDS material, smoking cessation material, promoting healthy traditions material, AIHCA brochure, and various reports generated by AIHCA.

CONSUMER HEALTH INFORMATION RESOURCE INSTITUTE *1-800-821-6671*
3030 Baltimore
Kansas City, MO 64108

MONTANA DEPARTMENT OF HEALTH AND ENVIRONMENTAL SCIENCES *1-406-444-2544 Executive office*
Cogswell Building
Helena, MT 59620

Purpose The organization addresses areas of public health in Montana, maternal and child health, handicapped children, dental health, disease control, communicable and chronic diseases, tuberculosis, venereal disease, cancer, heart disease, occupational health, environmental sanitation, air and water pollution, general sanitation, food and drug control, hospital facilities, health records and statistics, radiological health, health planning, and State Health Coordinating Council and administers preventive health and health services and maternal and child health block grant programs. It also answers inquiries, provides consulting services, and makes referrals.

Publications

Reports, directories, standards, and specifications.

NATIONAL HEALTH INFORMATION CENTER
Office of Disease Prevention and Health Promotion (ODPHP)
P.O. Box 1133
Washington, D.C. 20013-1133

1-301-565-4167 (in Maryland only)
1-800-336-4797
Weekdays: 9:00 A.M. to 5:00 P.M. EST

Purpose The Center was established in 1979 to provide referrals to sources on health-related issues. No referrals to physicians are made, but ODPHP will refer to self help groups. Gives toll-free numbers of organizations, if available. Provides callers with the organizations full addresses and phone numbers and/or refers questions to appropriate organizations so they can reply directly to requestors. Center components include health information resources in the federal government and locating funds for health promotion projects; It also responds to inquiries on rare diseases.

Publications

The Center produces directories, resource guides, and bibliographies on various health topics and disseminates many other ODPHP publications. Center publications include:

Healthfinders, a series of resource lists on current health concerns. Topics include health observances, toll-free numbers for health information, vitamins, health statistics, health risk appraisals, adolescent health, school health education, minority health, exercises for older Americans, family health, online health information, women's health, and health care financing.

Staying Healthy, a bibliography of health promotion materials, including an annotated list of pamphlets, manuals, posters, and audiovisuals produced by the U.S. Department of Health and Human Services.

NATIONAL INFORMATION SYSTEM FOR HEALTH RELATED SERVICES
University of South Carolina
Benson Building
Columbia, SC 29208

1-800-922-9234
1-800-922-1107,
(South Carolina only)

NATIONAL INSTITUTES OF HEALTH (NIH)
Office of Clinical Center Communications
Building 10, Room 1C255
Bethesda, MD 20892

1-301-496-2563

Publication

Behavior Patterns and Health, NIH Pub. No. 83-2625.

NORTH CAROLINA DEPARTMENT OF HUMAN RESOURCES CARELINE
325 N. Salisbury St.
Raleigh, NC 27611

1-800-662-7030 (North Carolina only)

OFFICE OF MINORITY HEALTH RESOURCE CENTER (OMH-RC)
P.O. Box 37337
Washington, D.C. 20013-7337

1-800-444-6472
Weekdays 9:00 A.M. to 5:00 P.M. EST

Purpose The Center maintains information on health-related resources available at the federal, state, and local levels that target Asians and Pacific Islanders, blacks, Hispanics/Latinos, and Native Americans. In addition to serving as a central source of minority health information, the OMH-RC works with the Office of Minority Health in identifying information gaps and in stimulating the development of resources where none exist. The activities of the OMH-RC concentrate on the following health priorities: cancer, chemical dependency, diabetes, heart disease/stroke, homicide/suicide and unintentional injury, and infant mortality. Information specialists refer requests to appropriate organizations, locate relevant materials, and identify sources of technical assistance. Bilingual staff are available to assist Spanish-speaking requestors.

Publications

Many reports on Task Force studies on black and minority health.

Closing the Gap Series, features publications produced by OMH-RC that summarize the minority health priority areas and associated risk factors. Titles in the series include

AIDS/HIV Infection and Minorities.

Cancer and Minorities.

Chemical Dependency and Minorities.

Diabetes and Minorities.

Health and Minorities U.S.

Heart Disease and Stroke and Minorities.

Homicide, Suicide, Unintentional Injuries & Minorities.

Infant Mortality and Minorities.

PENNSYLVANIA DEPARTMENT OF HEALTH
Health & Welfare Building, Room 929
6th & Commonwealth
Harrisburg, PA 17120

1-800-932-0912 (Pennsylvania only)

SOUTH DAKOTA TIE-LINE — *1-800-592-1865 (South Dakota only)*
Statewide Information Referral System
State Capitol
Pierre, SD 57501

VERMONT DEPARTMENT OF HEALTH — *1-800-642-3323 (Vermont only)*
60 Main Street
P.O. Box 70
Burlington, VT 05402

WISCONSIN CLEARINGHOUSE — *1-800-262-6243 (outside Wisconsin)*
University of Wisconsin
Dean of Students Office
Department K
P.O. Box 1468
Madison, WI 53701

HEALTH MAINTENANCE ORGANIZATIONS (HMOs)

Health Maintenance Organizations are group practices organized to provide complete care for patients on a prepaid basis. Patients or their employers provide care, at no extra charge or sometimes a nominal charge, for any illness or accident and preventive care such as checkups. The services covered by a particular HMO vary, depending upon the contract with patients.

HEALTH RESOURCES AND SERVICES ADMINISTRATION — *1-800-492-0359 English and Spanish (in Maryland only)*; *1-800-638-0742 English and Spanish (outside Maryland)*
Bureau of Health Maintenance
Organizations and Resources
Office of Health Facilities
5600 Fishers Lane
Rockville, MD 20857

HEARING

See also American Academy of Otolaryngology Head and Neck Surgery.

Deafness and other communication disorders affect more than one in ten individuals in the United States. Twenty-eight million persons are hearing-impaired. Contrary to popular belief, hearing loss is not restricted to the elderly.

Early warning signs of hearing loss include

- Failure to catch words or phrases
- Inability to follow conversations in a group as easily as do those around you
- Ability to better understand what a person is saying when you are facing him or her
- Frequently feeling that family and friends mumble instead of speaking clearly
- Hearing what seems to be distorted sounds
- Experiencing a running ear, pain, or irritation in the ear
- Suffering from dizziness, loss of balance, or head noises
- Your family complaining that you play the TV or radio too loudly
- You no longer hear normal household sounds such as the dripping of a faucet or the ringing of a doorbell

BETTER HEARING INSTITUTE — *1-800-424-8576 Helpline*

Box 1840 — *1-800-EAR WELL*

Washington, D.C. 20013

Purpose Professionals and others dedicated to helping persons with impaired hearing inform the public and the 20 million Americans who have impaired hearing about the nature of hearing loss and the availability of help.

NATIONAL ASSOCIATION FOR HEARING AND SPEECH ACTION — *1-301-897-8682*

10801 Rockville Pike — *1-800-638-8255*

Rockville, MD 20852

Purpose The Association seeks to provide information and referral services for people with speech, language, or hearing problems and their families. Refers to speech-language pathologists and audiologists within the requestor's geographic area. Also refers to self-help groups.

Publications

There are four brochures:

Hearing Impairment and the Audiologist.

How to Buy a Hearing Aid.

The National Association for Hearing and Speech Action Answers Questions About Assistive Listening Devices.

The National Association for Hearing and Speech Action Answers Questions About Noise and Hearing Loss.

NATIONAL INSTITUTE ON DEAFNESS AND OTHER COMMUNICATION DISORDERS (NIDOCD)
Clearing House
P.O. Box 37777
Washington, D.C. 20013-7777
1-301-496-7243
1-301-402-0252 TDD
Fax 1-301-402-0018

Publications

Hearing Loss: Hope Through Research, a 36-page booklet diagnosis and treatment of hearing loss.

Noise and Hearing Loss: A Consensus Statement, a 22-page booklet on noise-induced hearing loss.

NATIONAL INSTITUTES OF HEALTH (NIH)
Office of Clinical Center Communications
Building 10, Room 1C255
Bethesda, MD 20892
1-301-496-2563

Publication

Hearing Impairment: The Invisible Handicap, a videotape that can be borrowed.

OCCUPATIONAL HEARING SERVICE
Dial A Hearing Screen Test
P.O. Box 1880
Media, PA 19063
1-800-222-3277

TRIPOD GRAPEVINE (FOR HEARING IMPAIRED CHILDREN)
2901 North Keystone St.
Burbank, CA 91504
1-800-352-8888
1-800-346-8888 (California only)

HEARING AIDS

See also Deafness *and* Ears.

One in fifteen Americans suffers from hearing impairment. Our hearing begins to deteriorate at around age 30, and by the time we reach 65, one out of three of us could benefit from a hearing aid. Approximately four million people in the United States own a hearing aid.

INTERNATIONAL HEARING SOCIETY
Hearing Aid Helpline
20361 Middlebelt
Livonia, MI 48152
1-313-478-2610
1-800-521-5247

Purpose The Society seeks to provide a consumer service to the general public by supplying information and referrals to hearing instrument specialists in their area.

Publication
The World of Sound: Facts About Hearing Aids.

HEART

An estimated 68 million Americans have one or more forms of heart and blood vessel disease; it remains the nation's leading cause of death. Death rates from heart attack, stroke, and other cardiovascular diseases are declining. Advances in medical treatment and healthier life-styles have contributed to the decline, but there is still a long way to go and much that you can do to protect yourself and your family from this number one killer.

Major risk factors that can't be changed, according to The American Heart Association, are heredity, male sex, and increasing age. But *major risk factors that can be changed* are cigarette smoking, high blood pressure, blood cholesterol levels, diabetes, obesity, physical inactivity, and stress.

The following are the organizations and the information they provide to help you prevent heart disease and, if it occurs, to understand what you must do to live with it.

AMERICAN COLLEGE OF CARDIOLOGY *1-301-897-5400*
9111 Old Georgetown Road *1-800-253-4636 (in United States and Canada)*
Bethesda, MD 20814

Purpose The main purpose of the College of 19,300 cardiovascular specialists is to educate its members, but the staff will answer questions from the public. It does not make referrals, however.

Publications
What Is a Cardiologist? brochure describing the role of the cardiologist.
What Is a Pediatric Cardiologist?

AMERICAN HEART ASSOCIATION *1-214-373-6300*
7320 Greenville Ave.
Dallas, TX 75231-4599

Purpose The Association is a national voluntary health agency dedicated to the reduction of premature death or disability from cardiovascular diseases and stroke. This is accomplished through research support, medical education, public education, and community demonstration programs. It is interested in all aspects of cardiology and cardiovascular diseases; blood, cerebral, and kidney diseases in relation to the cardiovascular system; congenital heart disease; surgery; and prevention and control of heart disease.

Publications

GENERAL INFORMATION

Fact Sheet About Heart Attack, Stroke and Risk Factors of Cardiovascular Disease.

Heart and Blood Vessels—The Heart and Circulatory System and How They Work.

Heart Attack.

Heart Attack and Stroke: Signals and Action, a brochure that summarizes the impact that cardiovascular and cerebrovascular diseases have on the population in the United States, tells how to recognize and respond to heart attack and stroke. Also available in Spanish.

Heart Quiz, tests your knowledge about the heart and circulation.

Older Person's Guide to Cardiovascular Health

PREVENTION OF CORONARY HEART DISEASE

Coronary Risk Factor Statement for the American Public.

How to Make Your Heart Last a Lifetime.

How to Tell You're Having a Heart Attack—Early Warning Signs of a Heart Attack, and What To Do. Also available in Spanish.

DIET AND NUTRITION

About Your Heart and Diet.

Add More Potassium to Your Diet, a wallet card.

The American Heart Association Diet. An Eating Plan for Healthy Americans.

Cholesterol and Your Heart, a review of recent information. This pamphlet discusses the results of the coronary primary prevention trials, the implications of hyperlipidemia, and the AHA's dietary recommendations for the public. A fat and cholesterol content chart for selected foods is included.

Consumer Guide to Choosing and Using Nutrition Counseling for Cardiovascular Health.

Dining Out in New York City, tips on how to choose meals while dining out, and a survey of New York City restaurants that can accommodate special diets.

Eat Well But Eat Wisely, designed to reduce your risk of heart attack. A condensed review of the guidelines for a low-fat/low-cholesterol diet. Also available in Spanish.

Facts About Potassium.

A Guide to Losing Weight, a brief, easy-to-read pamphlet that gives the AHA's recommendations for reducing weight on a fat-controlled, nutritious eating plan. Also available in Spanish.

Nutrition for the Fitness Challenge.

Nutrition Labeling, food selection hints for a low-fat/low-cholesterol diet.

Nutritious Nibbles, a guide to healthy snacking.

Recipes for a Fat-Controlled Low Fat/Low Cholesterol Meals.

Salt, Sodium and Blood Pressure—Piecing Together the Puzzle.

Save Food Dollars and Help Your Heart.

Taking It Off.

Weight Control Guidance in Smoking Cessation.

HIGH BLOOD PRESSURE

About High Blood Pressure, a pamphlet that explains high blood pressure, controllable and non-controllable risk factors, the effects of high blood pressure on the body, and ways in which high blood pressure is treated. Also available in Spanish.

About High Blood Pressure in African Americans, a pamphlet, written jointly with the International Society on Hypertension in Blacks, helps African Americans understand what HBP is, the risk of developing it, and what can be done about it. It has also been approved by the Association of Black Cardiologists.

About High Blood Pressure in Children.

About Your Heart and Blood Pressure.

Buying and Caring for High Blood Pressure Equipment.

How You Can Help Your Doctor Treat Your High Blood Pressure—Now You're Cookin'—Healthful Recipes to Help Control HBP, a pamphlet containing helpful recipes to help control high blood pressure. The recipes are based on a fat-controlled, low-cholesterol meal plan recommended by medical experts.

Nutritious Nibbles: A Guide to Healthy Snacking, a pamphlet designed to help in making wise, nutritious, and enjoyable choices for snacking. Included are 12 recipe suggestions, hints on certain foods to avoid and those to include, and tips for enjoying a calorie-free break.

Salt, Sodium, and Blood Pressure—Piecing Together the Puzzle

Teenagers and High Blood Pressure.

Ten Commandments for the Person with High Blood Pressure, a wallet card. Also available in Spanish.

What Every Woman Should Know About High Blood Pressure.

What to Ask About High Blood Pressure.

SMOKING

About Your Heart & Smoking.

Calling It Quits, a self-help smoking cessation packet.

Children and Smoking (for Parents). Also available in Spanish.

Smoking and Heart Disease. Also available in Spanish.

Stub It & Stop It, a consumer guide to smoking cessation programs.

Weight Control Guidance in Smoking Cessation.

EXERCISE

About Your Heart & Exercise.

Aerobic Exercise Map of Manhattan.

Cycling for a Healthy Heart.

Dancing for a Healthy Heart.

"E" is for Exercise, a leaflet explaining the role of exercise in heart health. It depicts the types of exercise which might be recommended to promote cardiovascular fitness. It lists several factors one should consider before starting an exercise program. Also available in Spanish.

Exercise Diary, a booklet of grids and lined pages designed for the exerciser to use in setting goals and noting daily achievement.

Exercising Your Right to Know, a consumer guide to exercise testing and training centers.

Keeping the Beat.

Nutrition for the Fitness Challenge.

Roller Skating for a Healthy Heart.

Running for a Healthy Heart.

Swimming for a Healthy Heart.

Walking for a Healthy Heart.

RECOVERY AND REHABILITATION

After a Heart Attack, a booklet containing a description of the nature and result of a heart attack. It provides information to patients to help them deal with their feelings after a heart attack. Answers are given to commonly asked questions relative to life-style changes. Also available in Spanish.

Coronary Artery Bypass Graft Surgery.

Heart Surgery & Heart Catheterization.

Heart Valve Surgery.

Living with Your Pacemaker, a pamphlet for people who have a pacemaker. Includes explanation of how a pacemaker works, guidelines for understanding proper medications, and normal daily activities. A pacemaker identification card is included.

Sex and Heart Disease.

What You Should Know About Coronary Arteriography.

What You Should Know About P.T.C.A.

STROKE

Aphasia and the Family.

Body Language—How Your Body Warns You of an Impending Stroke, and What to Do About it.
Facts About Strokes. Also available in Spanish.
How Stroke Affects Behavior.
Recovering from a Stroke.
Stroke: The First Days.
Stroke: What It Is and What To Do.
Strokes—A Guide for the Family.

ABOUT CHILDREN

Abnormalities of Heart Rhythm: A Guide for Parents.
About High Blood Pressure in Children.
Children and Smoking (for parents). Also in Spanish.
Dental Care for Children with Congenital Heart Disease.
Feeding Infants with Congenital Heart Disease.
If Your Child Has Congenital Heart Defect.
Innocent Heart Murmurs in Children. Also available in Spanish.
Kawasaki Disease.
Teenagers and High Blood Pressure.
You, Your Child and Rheumatic Fever.

FOR CHILDREN

About Your Heart & Bloodstream.
The Case of the Sudden Sickness, a comic book about smoking.
Circulatory System, a diagram.
Cycling for a Healthy Heart.
Dancing for a Healthy Heart.
Roller Skating for a Healthy Heart.
Running for a Healthy Heart.
Swimming for a Healthy Heart.
Your Heart & How it Works, a diagram. It includes a word game on the back.

MISCELLANEOUS

Anticoagulants, Your Physician & You.
Aspirin and Your Heart.
Bacterial Endocarditis Wallet Card, for the patient with rheumatic fever, valvular disease, or congenital heart disease who needs protection from bacterial endocarditis when undergoing medical or dental treatment.
Cardiocard, a medical identification card from the World Health Organization. Available in several languages.
Facts About Congestive Heart Failure.

First Aid for Choking, wallet card that shows proper emergency action to follow for an adult conscious and unconscious choking victim. Its convenient size allows interested persons to have this information readily available.

Mitral Valve Prolapse.

Question and Answer About Chelation Therapy.

YOUR HEART DURING PREGNANCY

Understanding Angina.

Varicose Veins.

POSTERS

On smoking:

Come to Where the Air Is Fresh.

No Smoking.

Now Call It "Quits."

Pregnant Woman Smoking.

Set Good Example, (for the family with young children (set of 2).

Thank You for Not Smoking Posters (set of 2).

Thank You for Not Smoking Table Tents.

On blood pressure:

Announcements for a Blood Pressure Screening (Set of 2)

Blood Pressure Up? Don't Let It Get You Down.

Feelin' Great! Have Your Blood Pressure Checked.

Scale Down.

Take Your Medications.

Take Your Pills Along (When Traveling).

What Goes Up Must Come Down.

On exercise:

Exercise Is Wise.

Love Your Heart.

Target Heart Rate.

On miscellaneous:

Culinary Hearts, kitchen poster.

Do Something, CPR poster.

Don't Give These Signals a Second Thought—Don't Learn These Warning Signs the Hard Way. Eat Fast . . . Eat Smart.

February Is the Month for Hearts.

How to Tell You're Having a Heart Attack. Also available in Spanish.

Never Forget Who You're Saving Your Heart For.

ARIZONA HEART INSTITUTE & FOUNDATION (AHI&F)
2632 N. 20th Street
Phoenix, AZ 85006

1-602-266-2200 Ext. 661
1-800-345-HART (4278)
Weekdays 8 A.M. to 5 P.M. MST

Purpose The AHI&F promotes the prevention, diagnosis, and least invasive treatment of heart disease. The trained staff is on call to answer questions on all aspects of heart and blood vessel disease. Also provides information on diet and fitness.

Publications
Offers the following fact sheets:
Alternatives to Surgery.
Aneurysms.
Arizona Heart Institute.
Bacterial Endocarditis.
Cardiac Catheterization/Coronary Angioplasty.
Cardiac Medications.
Care of Your Legs & Feet.
Carotid Artery Disease & Stroke.
Chelation.
Children's Snacks.
Congenital Heart Disease.
Congestive Heart Failure.
Coronary Artery Bypass Surgery.
Dining Out.
Elevated Lipid Management.
Exercise.
Food Labeling.
Heart Attack/Angina.
Heart Disease.
Heart Health Diet.
Heart Transplantation.
How to Live to be 100.
Hypertension.
Irregular Heartbeats.
Marfan's Syndrome.
Mitral Valve Prolapse.
Pacemakers.
Peripheral Vascular Disease.
Risk Factors of Cardiovascular Disease.
Smoking.
Stress.
Valvular Heart Disease.
Vein Disorders.
Weight Loss.
Women & Heart Disease.

HEALTH AND HUMAN SERVICES, DEPARTMENT OF; PUBLIC HEALTH SERVICE; NATIONAL INSTITUTES OF HEALTH; NATIONAL HEART, LUNG, AND BLOOD INSTITUTE
Communications and Public Information Branch
Bldg 31, Room 4A 21
Bethesda, MD 20892

1-301-496-4236
Information office
1-301-951-3260
Information center

Purpose The Communications and Public Information Branch conducts research and training relating to the causes, prevention, diagnosis, and treatment of diseases of the heart and circulation, of chronic lung diseases such as emphysema and bronchitis, and of certain blood diseases such as sickle cell disease and hemophilia; blood resources; and health effects of cholesterol and smoking. It has a data bank on the Institute's research and training grants and awards, and develops the High Blood Pressure subfile in the Combined Health Information Data Base. The Branch also has access to the DIALOG, BRS, and NEXIS computerized database and has an in-house online catalog of programmatic materials in the areas of high blood pressure, cholesterol, smoking, and blood resource. Answers phone inquiries.

Publications

Informational and Educational Materials, a catalog listing leaflets, booklets, and other information/education materials is available on request from the Public Inquiries and Reports Branch.

MENDED HEARTS, INC.
7320 Greenville Ave.
Dallas, TX 75231

1-214-706-1442

Purpose

An affiliation of persons throughout the United States who suffer from heart disease, Mended Hearts, Inc., has chapters in many states. Answers inquiries; and provides encouragement and other services to persons anticipating or recovering from heart surgery as well as to their families. Specially trained Mended Hearts Accredited Visitors strive to resolve troubling questions, to be of moral support, and to help make the time through surgery and recovery easier for the patient and the family.

Publications

Getting to the Heart of the Matter, a brochure describing Mended Hearts services.

Heartbeat, a quarterly journal for members and subscribers. Contains articles of interest to heart disease patients, families, and others interested in diet, exercise, and new technologies.

Heart to Heart, a brochure describing the chapters and the services offered.

To the Family of the Heart Surgery Patient, a brochure describing services to help patients and their families.

NATIONAL CENTER FOR CARDIAC INFORMATION (NCCI) *1-703-764-0060*
P.O. Box 271
Burke, VA 22015-0271

Purpose The National Center for Cardiac Information, a nonprofit organization and part of the United States Policy Committee educational foundation, was established to provide timely and useful preventive health information to potential victims of heart attacks and strokes. NCCI's primary goal is to provide the general public with information and advice on how diet and exercise can benefit the heart. NCCI plans include representing the public by lobbying for more variety in low-fat, low-cholesterol foods; challenging the major supermarket chains to lower their prices on heart healthy foods; improving labeling; adding special aisles for shopping convenience; undertaking a public service advertising campaign for school-aged children; and sponsoring information campaigns targeting young mothers.

NATIONAL HEART, LUNG, AND BLOOD INSTITUTE (NHLBI) *1-301-496-4236*
Building 31, Room 4A-21
9000 Rockville Pike
Bethesda, MD 20892

Purpose The Institute was established in 1948 as the National Heart Institute; its name was changed by legislative mandate to the National Heart, Lung, and Blood Institute. Its primary responsibility is the scientific investigation of heart, blood vessel, lung, and blood diseases. The Institute oversees resources and research, demonstration, prevention, education, control, and training activities in these fields. The program emphasizes the prevention and control of heart, lung, and blood diseases and education concerning these diseases through more rapid transfer of knowledge into the mainstream of clinical medicine and personal health practices. Limited quantities of a variety of topical pamphlets and other publications are available free of charge upon request. Inquiries related to high blood pressure, cholesterol, smoking, asthma, and blood resource (blood banking, blood transfusion), as well as any information requests associated with cardiovascular disease prevention and heart health promotion, are handled by the National Heart, Lung, and Blood Institute Education Programs' Information Center under Public Law 96-538, Health Programs Extension Act of 1980.

Publications

Check Your Blood I.Q., NIH Pub. No. 88-2991.

Check Your Weight and Heart Disease I.Q., NIH Pub. No. 90-3034, a 2-page, 11-question true/false quiz that addresses the independent relationship of obesity/overweight to coronary heart disease as well as its relationship to high blood pressure, high blood cholesterol, and smoking habits.

The Healthy Heart Handbook for Women, NIH Pub. No. 89-2720.

Heart and Heart/Lung Transplant (Facts About), NIH Pub. No. 90-2990.

Heart Attacks, NIH Pub. No. 86-2700.

High Blood Pressure and What You Can Do About It.

Mitral Valve Prolapse (NHLBI Facts About).

Momentum Toward Health, NIH Pub. No. 85-2353.

Nutrition and Your Health: Dietary Guidelines for Americans Home & Garden Bulletin No. 232, a 2-page pamphlet containing seven guidelines that answer the questions regarding what Americans should eat to stay healthy. Prepared jointly by the U.S. Department of Agriculture and the U.S. Department of Health and Human Services.

Play Your Cards Right . . . Stay Young at Heart, NIH Pub. No. NN405, a supplement to the *Guidelines*, this pamphlet contains 15 new heart healthy recipes.

Step to the Beat of a Healthy Heart, a poster.

Test Your Healthy Heart I.Q., NIH Pub. No. 88-2724. Also available in Spanish, NIH Pub. No. 85-2923.

Treat Yourself Right, a poster.

NATIONAL HEART, LUNG, AND BLOOD INSTITUTE *1-301-951-3260*
EDUCATION PROGRAMS
Information Center
Information Specialist
4733 Bethesda Avenue, Suite 530
Bethesda, MD 20814

Purpose The National Heart, Lung, and Blood Institute Education Programs' Information Center was established in 1986 as a source of information and materials on cholesterol and smoking, two major risk factors for cardiovascular health. In 1987, it was merged with the National High Blood Pressure Education Program. Two new programs, the National Blood Resource Education Program and the National Asthma Education Program, have also been established. Services include dissemination of public education materials, programmatic and scientific information for health professionals, materials on worksite health, and response to information requests. The Cholesterol, High Blood Pressure, and Smoking Education Database is a subfile on the Combined Health Information Database (CHID) available on BRS Information Technologies. The Center is a service of the National Heart, Lung, and Blood Institute of the National Institutes of Health.

NATIONAL INSTITUTES OF HEALTH *1-301-496-2563*
Office of Clinical Center Communications
Building 10, Room 1C255
Bethesda, MD 20892

Publication
Risk of Heart Disease, NIH Pub. No. 89-2985.

SCHERING-PLOUGH CORPORATION/KEY PHARMACEUTICALS *1-908-298-4000*
2000 Galloping Hill Road
Kenilworth, NJ 07033

Publications

A Message For You, information regarding the treatment of angina, including the use of the NITO-DUR (nitroglycerin) transdermal infusion system.

Your Doctor Says You Need a Potassium Supplement, overview with regard to the need for potassium and/or a potassium supplement (K-DUR 20).

HEARTBURN

Heartburn is characterized by a mild to severe burning sensation in the upper abdomen or beneath the breastbone, usually resulting from backingup of stomach contents into the throat. Heartburn typically occurs after a heavy meal containing fatty foods. It is usually more pronounced when you are lying down or are sitting with your feet slightly elevated and is relieved by sitting up.

NATIONAL INSTITUTE OF DIABETES AND DIGESTIVE AND KIDNEY DISEASES (NIDDKD) *1-301-499-3583*
Building 31, Room 9A04
Bethesda, MD 20892

Publication

Heartburn, NIH Pub. No. 86-882.

HEMOCHROMATOSIS

An overload of iron in the body associated with tissue injury is known as hemochromatosis. Symptoms may include:

- Fatigue
- Arthritis
- Diabetes
- Heart irregularities
- Enlarged liver and/or cirrhosis
- Decreased libido, early loss of periods
- Tan not due to sun exposure

HEMOCHROMATOSIS RESEARCH FOUNDATION, INC. *1-518-489-0972*
P.O. Box 8569
Albany, NY 12208

Purpose The Hemochromatosis Research Foundation, Inc., was formed to increase the awareness of the public, the medical community, and the government that hereditary hemochromatosis is one of the most common genetic disorders; to encourage routine screenings for hemochromatosis in all individuals, especially those with arthritis, diabetes, heart irregularities and failure, and liver diseases; and to solicit funds for research. The Foundation estimates 1.6 million Americans are afflicted with the disorder and remain undiagnosed and that another 25 to 32 million are carriers. The Foundation sponsors Family Teaching Conferences at teaching institutions, periodic teleconferences for both patients and physicians, and periodic international conferences for researchers and physicians.

Publications

Send a stamped, self-addressed, envelope for
Hereditary (Genetic or Idiopathic) Hemochromatosis.
Some Facts About Hemochromatosis.

HEMODIALYSIS

See Kidney.

HEMOPHILIA

Hemophilia is the most common of the bleeding diseases. It is a condition in which there is a reduction in the amount of a protein called antihemophilic globulin, or Factor VIII, in the blood. The factor is necessary for blood clotting. In the United States, about 1 male in 10,000 has hemophilia.

NATIONAL HEMOPHILIA FOUNDATION *212-431-8541*
110 Greene St., Suite 406 *1-800-424-2634 or 1-800-42-HANDI*
New York, NY 10012 *Fax 1-212-431-0906*

Purpose The Foundation provides information on hemophilia and AIDS/HIV to NHF chapters and to hemophilia treatment center professionals nationwide, as well as to people with hemophilia, their family members and caregivers, and others in need of information. HANDI has at its disposal a growing collection of materials on hemophilia and AIDS/HIV from a variety of sources. Referrals are made to physicians and self-help groups.

Publications

Audio and audiovisual materials and posters.
HANDI Quarterly, a newsletter that reports on the projects and activities of the organization.
Publications for the person with hemophilia, family, and community (multilingual).
Resource publications.
A 23-page resource listing, including publications for the hemophilia care provider.
Single copies of all items listed are free of charge upon request.

HEMORRHOIDS

Hemorrhoids are dilated, overstretched, varicose veins in and around the rectal opening. Symptoms due to hemorrhoids include bleeding, protrusion of the veins, and pain.

NATIONAL INSTITUTE OF DIABETES AND DIGESTIVE AND KIDNEY DISEASES (NIDDKD) *1-301-499-3583*
Building 31, Room 9A04
Bethesda, MD 20892

Publication

Hemorrhoids, NIH Pub. No. 89-3021.

HERPES

See also under American Social Health Association.

Herpes simplex is a recurrent viral infection characterized by the appearance on the skin or mucous membranes of single or multiple clusters of small vesicles, filled with clear fluid, on slightly raised inflammatory bases. Herpes simplex 2 virus, which is commonly referred to just as "herpes," has been transmitted through sexual contact to an estimated 30 million Americans. Half of the people who carry the virus never get the genital blisters that are the major symptoms of the infection, so they may not know they can transmit it. "Shingles" and "cold sores" are produced by other herpes viruses.

NATIONAL HERPES HOTLINE *1-919-361-8488*
Weekdays, 9 A.M.–7 P.M. EST

NATIONAL INSTITUTE OF ALLERGY AND INFECTIOUS DISEASES (NIAID) *1-301-496-5717*
Building 31, Room 7A32
Bethesda, MD 20892

Publication

Genital Herpes, NIH Pub. No. 84-2005. Also available in Spanish, NIH Pub. No. 84-656.

NATIONAL INSTITUTES OF HEALTH (NIH) *1-301-496-2563*
Office of Clinical Center Communications
Building 10, Room 1C255
Bethesda, MD 20892

Publication

Herpes, NIH Pub. No. 85-0858.

SCHERING-PLOUGH CORPORATION/KEY PHARMACEUTICALS *1-908-298-4000*
2000 Galloping Hill Road
Kenilworth, NJ 07033

Publication

Herpes Zoster (Shingles).

HIGH BLOOD PRESSURE

It is estimated that nearly 60 million Americans have high blood pressure. Physicians generally diagnose high blood pressure when an otherwise healthy adult has consistent readings above 140/90. The upper number in a blood pressure reading is a measurement made when the heart is contracting, the systolic pressure. The lower number in a blood pressure reading is recorded when the heart is at rest, called the diastolic pressure.

LEDERLE LABORATORIES *1-201-831-4692*
Public and Government Affairs
One Cyanamid Plaza
Wayne, NJ 07470

Publication

Keeping Fit: Learning to Live with Your High Blood Pressure, a 36-page booklet giving an overview of the problem, the medications prescribed, and ways to increase your heart power. A glossary is also included.

NATIONAL CENTER FOR RESEARCH RESOURCES (NCRR) *1-301-496-5545*
Westwood Building, Room 857
Bethesda, MD 20892

Publication

Advances in Hypertension Research

NATIONAL HEART, LUNG, AND BLOOD INSTITUTE (NHLBI) *1-301-496-4236*
Building 31, Room 4A21
Bethesda, MD 20892

Publications

Blacks and High Blood Pressure, NIH Pub. No. 87-2024, an 8-page booklet that describes high blood pressure, its prevalence among blacks, the need for treatment, and the role of the patient's family. Written for black consumers and blacks with high blood pressure.

Questions About Weight, Salt, and High Blood Pressure, NIH Pub. No. 88-1459, describes what is known about the relationship between certain diet changes and high blood pressure. Written for people newly diagnosed with hypertension and their families.

Their Future Is in Your Hands—Treat Your High Blood Pressure Every Day, a poster that depicts Hispanic children with the text in Spanish.

Three Good Reasons to Control Your High Blood Pressure, a poster that shows "person-on-the-street" interviews to motivate people with high blood pressure to adhere to their treatment.

Working Group Report on Ambulatory Blood Pressure Monitoring, NIH Pub. No. 90-3028 (consensus of experts on monitoring), a 21-page report that examines the state of the technology of ambulatory blood pressure monitoring. Topics covered include equipment and standards, ambulatory blood pressure recording, clinical utility of 24-hour monitoring, and cost considerations. The report concludes with the working group's recommendations.

Working Group Report on High Blood Pressure in Pregnancy, (consensus of experts on the subject), NIH Pub. No. 90-3029, a 38-page report that provides guidance to physicians in managing hypertensive patients who become pregnant and managing pregnant patients who become hypertensive (the pregnancy-specific condition is termed preeclampsia).

Working Group Report on Management of Patients with Hypertension and High Blood Cholesterol, (consensus of experts on the subject), NIH Pub. No. 90-2361, a 30-page report designed to guide doctors in managing patients with multiple cardiovascular risk factors, placing a special emphasis on hypertension and high blood cholesterol.

In Spanish:

Presion Alto: Lo Que Usted y su Familia Deben Saber (High Blood Pressure: Things You and Your Family Should Know), NIH Pub. No. 88-2025, an 8-page booklet that describes what high pressure is, how it is treated, and the role of the patient's family.

NATIONAL INSTITUTES OF HEALTH (NIH) *1-301-496-2563*
Office of Clinical Center Communications
Building 10, Room 1C255
Bethesda, MD 20892

Publication

High Blood Pressure.

SCHERING-PLOUGH CORPORATION/KEY PHARMACEUTICALS *1-908-298-4000*
2000 Galloping Hill Road
Kenilworth, NJ 07033

Publication

Understanding High Blood Pressure, answers such questions as "What is blood pressure and specifically high blood pressure?" "How do you know you have high blood pressure?" "What can you do to minimize your risks?"

HOME CARE

The aging population, one day surgery, and out-of-hospital medical services contribute to more and more patients being cared for at home. Most patients are happier at home. If they require sophisticated medical care, help is available.

NATIONAL ASSOCIATION FOR HOME CARE (NAHC) *1-202-547-7424*
519 C Street, N.E, *Fax 1-202-547-3540*
Washington, D.C. 20002-5809

Purpose NAHC is a nonprofit trade association that lobbies on behalf of the home care agencies across the country. The organization has been representing home care providers for the past ten years. Direct access to the regulatory, legislative, and legal experts on staff is the most touted benefit. NAHC does not refer consumers to home care providers but will answer questions.

VISITING NURSE ASSOCIATIONS OF AMERICA *1-800-426-2547*
3801 E. Florida Avenue, Suite 206
Denver, CO 80210

Purpose The Association provides information on home health care services, physical therapy, occupational therapy, speech, and general nursing. It will provide referrals to one of the 426 organizations in your locale.

Publication

Brochure.

WELL SPOUSE FOUNDATION *1-619-673-9043*
P.O. Box 28876 *1-914-357-8513*
San Diego, CA 92198-0876

Purpose More than 7 million healthy Americans have spouses who are chronically ill. For the well spouses, life is a constant struggle against emotional debilitation, physical exhaustion, and often financial destitution. The Well Spouse Foundation provides emotional support for spouses and partners of the chronically ill. Inform medical profession and public of the well caretaker's needs. Advocate for long-term care insurance and home health care and against spousal impoverishment.

Publication
Brochure About WSF and How to Join.

HOMEOPATHIC MEDICINE

The name is derived from the Greek words, *homeo* for "alike" and *pathos* for "feeling," "suffering," or "disease." Homeopathy is a system of therapy developed by Samuel Hahnemann based on the law of "similia." that is, likes are cured by likes. Homeopaths believe that a medicinal substance that can evoke certain symptoms in healthy individuals may be effective in the treatment of illnesses having symptoms closely resembling those produced by the substance.

HOMEOPATHIC EDUCATIONAL SERVICES *1-510-649-0294*
2124 Kittredge St., Room Q40
Berkeley, CA 94704

Purpose Homeopathic Educational Services provides a free comprehensive catalog of books, tapes, and general information on homeopathic medicine and operates both a mail-order service and a retail store. No referrals are made by phone.

HOSPICE

Although most Americans are born and die in hospitals, there is a growing movement—both economical and societal—to experience dying amid an atmosphere of empathy and love. The hospice (from the Latin name for a "host" or "guest," *hospes*) provides a centralized program of palliative and supportive services to dying persons and their families. Psychological, social, and spiritual services are rendered by an interdisciplinary team of professionals and volunteers who are available at home and in inpatient settings.

CHILDREN'S HOSPICE INTERNATIONAL (CHI) *1-703-684-0330*
901 N. Washington St., Suite 200 *1-800-2-4-CHILD*
Alexandria, VA 22314-2502

Purpose A nonprofit organization which has received project funding from the U.S. Department of Health and Human Services, Division of Maternal and Child Health, CHI provides a support system and resource bank sharing expertise and information with health care professionals, families, and the network of organizations within communities that offer hospice care to terminally ill children. Referrals are made to self-help groups, hospice programs, and other related groups or programs.

Publications
Publications list. Charges for publications.

HOSPICE EDUCATION INSTITUTE *1-800-331-1620 HospiceLink*
5 Essex Square, Suite 3-B
P.O. Box 713
Essex, CT 06426-0713

Purpose The Institute provides national information and referral service to hospices and palliative care services throughout the United States. It answers general questions on principles and good practices in terminal care and offers "sympathetic listening" to persons who wish to discuss problems relating to terminal illness or bereavement.

Publications
Bibliography on terminal care and bereavement.
Brochures describing hospice care and HospiceLink.
Textbook on symptom control.

NATIONAL HOSPICE ORGANIZATION (NHO) *1-800-658-8898*
1901 North Moore St., Suite 901
Arlington, VA 22209

Purpose NHO is devoted entirely to hospice. Services to members include informational updates, technical assistance, access to helpful publications, lobbying, and access to conferences. It provides general information on hospice philosophy and referrals to local hospice programs and refers to local hospice programs.

Publications
About Hospice, a scriptographic booklet outlining hospice services.

The Basics of Hospice, a brochure outlining philosophy, services and payment.

Guide to the Nation's Hospices, a comprehensive listing of all hospices. There is a substantial cost to purchase the entire book, but NHO will mail out photocopied pages of specified areas for free.

NATIONAL INSTITUTE FOR JEWISH HOSPICE — *1-800-446-4448*, *1-213-HOSPICE*
ASB/1 Bldg., Suite 652
8723 Alden Dr.
Los Angeles, CA 90048

Purpose Headquartered in Los Angeles and New York with support groups in major cities, the Institute designs ways to serve terminally ill Jewish patients and their relatives by training caregivers of all faiths. The emphasis is on developing humane palliative strategies that are tailored to the needs of Jewish patients.

HOSPITALS

Hospitals are providing less in-patient services and more out-patient services than in the past. Hospitals are characterized by the type of services provided, length of hospital stay, type of health care providers and as teaching or nonteaching institutions. The two basic divisions are the voluntary, short-stay general community hospitals and nonfederal, long-term hospitals. Most voluntary hospitals are community institutions that are non-profit associations of citizens who form a corporation that includes trustees responsible for the hospital's actions.

NATIONAL CENTER FOR RESEARCH RESOURCES — *1-301-496-5545*
Westwood Bldg, Room 857
Bethesda, MD 20892

Publication
General Clinical Research Centers—Patient Information.

HUNTINGTON'S CHOREA

A progressive hereditary disease usually beginning in middle age and characterized by jerky movements and progressive intellectual deterioration.

HUNTINGTON'S DISEASE SOCIETY OF AMERICA (HDSA) — *1-212-242-1968*, *1-800-345-HDSA*
140 W. 22nd St., 6th Floor
New York, NY 10011-2420

Purpose The Society is the only national voluntary agency providing support and services to people with Huntington's disease (HD) and their families. HDSA is dedicated to both improving the lives of people with HD and their families and to finding a cure for HD. The Society's programs include research, patient and family services, education, and advocacy. Support is given to chapters and self-help groups.

The Society will refer to health care professionals, nursing homes, and other specialized services.

Publications

The Society has books, articles, and pamphlets. It also has a collection of videos for rental.

HYDROCEPHALUS

Hydrocephalus is a condition in which fluid builds up in the head due to an obstruction of the canals that circulate the cerebrospinal fluid around the brain and spinal cord. Most frequently, it is a congenital defect. Acquired causes include brain hemorrhage, cyst, tumor, and infection. Hydrocephalus affects about 1 in 500 children born, and, less frequently, adolescents and mature adults.

GUARDIANS OF HYDROCEPHALUS RESEARCH FOUNDATION — *1-718-743-GHRF*
2618 Avenue Z — *Fax 1-718-934-3254*
Brooklyn, NY 11235-2023

Purpose The GHRF's aim is to educate the general public about hydrocephalus (water on the brain) and disseminate information for a better understanding of hydrocephalus. The organization maintains a free evaluation center (NYUMC) to help the afflicted deal with their problems and helps to fund a research program. Refers to physicians and self-help groups through the assistance of the medical advisory board.

Publications

An Introduction to Hydrocephalus, a booklet written in English and Spanish, explaining hydrocephalus, the shunt, and its effects.

HYDROCEPHALUS ASSOCIATION — *1-415-776-4713*
2040 Polk Street, Room 342
San Francisco, CA 94109

Purpose A nonprofit organization founded in 1984 by parents of children and young adults with hydrocephalus, the Association provides support, education, resources, and advocacy to parents and professionals. The members strongly believe that the most effective long-term care program for individuals with hydrocephalus depends on the creation of an effective health care team. It will refer to pediatric neurosurgeons.

Publications

About Hydrocephalus, a book for parents.
Directory of Pediatric Neurosurgeons.

Hydrocephalus Association, a brochure.
Hydrocephalus Association Newsletter.
Resource Guide.

NATIONAL HYDROCEPHALUS FOUNDATION *1-815-467-6548*
400 N. Michigan Ave., Suite 1102
Chicago, IL 60611-4102

Purpose The Foundation's mission is to familiarize the public with the term hydrocephalus, to remove the stigma from those who have the condition, and to define specific problems that parents of children with hydrocephalus encounter and to resolve them as best as possible. The Foundation also disseminates information and advocates the health insurance coverage and resources to aid in the treatment of hydrocephalus.

Publications
Bibliography.
Life-Line, a quarterly newsletter.
National Hydrocephalus Foundation, a brochure.

HYPERACTIVITY

See Attention Deficit Disorder.

HYPNOSIS

There is much misinformation about hypnosis. The physical and mental state of the hypnotized individual is a matter of speculation. The consensus is that the therapeutic benefits from hypnotism depend upon the expectations and needs of the patient, the ability and expectations of the doctor, and the interpersonal relationship or rapport between patient and doctor.

AMERICAN SOCIETY OF CLINICAL HYPNOSIS *1-708-297-3317*
22000 East Devon Avenue, Suite 291 *Fax 1-708-297-7309*
Des Plaines, IL 60018-4534

Purpose The Society seeks to advance the use of hypnosis in clinical practice and to educate health care professionals in the clinical uses of the modality. Referrals are made to persons sending a stamped, self-addressed envelope for a referral list.

HYPOGLYCEMIA

A deficiency of sugar in the blood may be life threatening in diabetics, but it is a controversial diagnosis in others. Often suspected of causing symptoms such as fatigue, lethargy, loss of libidio, dry skin, and depression, many physicians believe true hypoglycemia is a rare condition. Others believe that it is underdiagnosed and that the condition may exist even if conventional blood tests do not detect it.

NATIONAL HYPOGLYCEMIA ASSOCIATION (NHA) *1-201-670-1189*
P.O. Box 120
Ridgewood, NJ 07451

Purpose The aim of the organization is to be informative, educational, and supportive to hypoglycemics and their families. Makes referrals to support groups and to specialists in hypoglycemia in a requestor's locale, if possible.

Publication

Hypoglycemia—This Is What It's All About, by Leonore L. Cohen, founder and director of NHA.

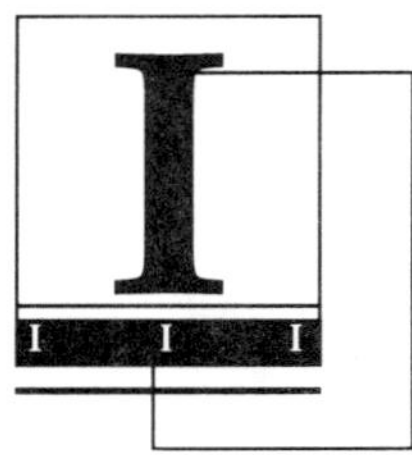

IMMUNOLOGY

New understanding of how the body protects itself against disease and injury is leading to new treatments that will alleviate ills from birth defects to cancer. With newly detailed pictures of molecules that sit on the surfaces of cells, scientists are hopeful that they will be able to devise strategies against the more than 40 diseases that result when the immune system mistakenly turns against the body, including arthritis and lupus.

AMERICAN ACADEMY OF ALLERGY AND IMMUNOLOGY *1-800-822-2762*
611 East Wells St.
Milwaukee,WI 53202

Publication

Facts About Immune Thrombocytopenic Purpura (ITP) (Facts About), NIH Pub. No. 90-2114.

NATIONAL INSTITUTE OF ALLERGY AND INFECTIOUS DISEASES (NIAID) *1-301-496-5717*
Building 31, Room 7A32
9000 Rockville Pike
Bethesda, MD 20205

Publication

Understanding The Immune System, NIH Pub. No. 88-529, a 36-page pamphlet describing the complex network of specialized cells and organs that make up the human immune system. It explains how the system works to fight off disease caused by invading agents, such as bacteria and viruses, and how it sometimes malfunctions, resulting in a variety of diseases from allergies, to arthritis, to cancer. It was developed by the National Institute of Allergy and Infectious Diseases and printed by the NCI.

IMPOTENCE

See Sex Therapy.

INCEST

See Abuse.

INCONTINENCE

See Urinary Incontinence *and* Kidney Foundation.

INFECTIOUS DISEASES

See also Laboratory Topics.

The control and prevention of infectious diseases has traditionally been a primary health goal. Systematic reporting of various diseases in the United States began in 1874. There are basically two major types of infectious agents—viruses and bacteria. Viruses come in many tiny shapes and sizes and do their dirty work by invading the cell and taking over the reproductive mechanisms. Bacteria also come in many shapes and are everywhere. Some are harmless and some are lethal.

CENTERS FOR DISEASE CONTROL (CDC) *1-404-332-4555*
1600 Clifton Road, N.E.
Atlanta, GA 30333

Purpose Originally established as the Communicable Disease Center, CDC continues to maintain its expertise in infectious disease control but now has the broader mission of preventing all unnecessary morbidity and mortality. Newer programs at CDC include environmental health, prevention of occupational disease and accidents, and promotion of health through education and information. You can access information on various diseases by calling the number listed and selecting an option on a touch-tone phone. Also supports the National AIDS information clearinghouse. See under AIDS.

NATIONAL FOUNDATION FOR INFECTIOUS DISEASES *1-301-656-0003*
4733 Bethesda Ave., Suite 750
Bethesda, MD 20814

Purpose This non-profit, nongovernmental organization was founded in 1973 to support research into the prevention of and education about infectious diseases.

Publication

The Double Helix, newsletter about developments in combatting infectious diseases such as AIDs, TB, vaginal yeast infections, and immune disorders.

NATIONAL INSTITUTE OF ALLERGY AND INFECTIOUS DISEASES (NIAID) *1-301-496-5717*
Building 31, Room 7A32
Bethesda, MD 20205

Publications

At the Edge of Life: An Introduction to Viruses, NIH Pub. No. 80-433.
Bacterial Meningitis, NIH Pub. No. 84-1439.

INFERTILITY

See also Endometriosis.

Infertility is defined as the inability to become pregnant after one year of trying or to carry a pregnancy to term. Five million American couples are trying to start families but they cannot. There are many new options, thanks to technological developments such as *in vitro* fertilization and sperm banks.

AMERICAN COLLEGE OF OBSTETRICIANS AND GYNECOLOGISTS (ACOG) *1-202-638-5577*
409 12th Street, S.W.
Washington, D.C. 20024-2188

Purpose With a membership of more than 29,000 physicians specializing in obstetrics-gynecologic care, the American College of Obstetricians and Gynecologists serves as a strong advocate for quality health care for women; maintaining the highest standards of clinical practice and continuing education for its members; promoting patient education and stimulating patient understanding, and involvement in, medical care; and increasing awareness among its members and the public of the changing issues facing women's health care. Responds to specific questions and refers to physicians and associations.

Publication

Contraception, a pamphlet that describes how the various contraceptives work.

The Pap Test, a pamphlet that explains the procedure and its value and includes a glossary.

Patient Education, an order form for the many other educational pamphlets and books provided by the College.

Premenstrual Syndrome, a pamphlet that describes a group of physical or behavioral changes that some women go through before their menstrual periods begin.

AMERICAN FERTILITY SOCIETY
2140 Eleventh Ave. South, Suite 200
Birmingham, Al 35205-2800

1-205-933-8494
Fax 205-930-9904

Purpose The Society is the world's largest and fastest-growing subspecialty group in the medical field. Some 10,500 physicians and scientists from every state and more than 118 foreign countries belong. The organization provides current information on reproductive health. Referrals are made to physicians specializing in infertility and to self-help groups.

RESOLVE, INC.
1310 Broadway
Somerville, MA 02144-1731

1-617-623-1156 Business office
1-617-623-0744 Helpline

Purpose RESOLVE's purpose is to serve the needs of the infertile population and allied professionals with information, education, and advocacy. It provides a telephone helpline with referrals to physicians, IVF clinics, local chapters, and local support groups.

Publication

RESOLVE: When You're Wishing for a Baby, a brochure on the organization and the services available.

A list of books, articles, and fact sheets for sale.

SERONO SYMPOSIA, USA
100 Longwater Circle
Norwell, MA 02061

1-617-982-9000
1-800-283-8088
Fax 1-617-982-9481

Purpose This organization assists with the education of people experiencing infertility and provides patient literature and listings of RESOLVE chapters nationwide and listings of educational consumer symposia held nationwide.

Publications

ART: Assisted Reproductive Technologies, by Ricardo H. Asch, M.D., and Richard P. Marrs, M.D., a booklet that describes several different techniques or procedures now available to help couples achieve pregnancy after other surgical and hormonal methods have failed. This booklet describes many aspects of the ARTs, from patient selection to the procedural elements of and variations among these techniques, and also provides some recent statistical data.

Infertility and Insurance Brochure, 1992 Update, by Janet Stroup Fox, a guide for advocates of expanded insurance coverage for infertility treatment and for the lay public who may not be aware that lack of coverage is a pressing problem. This brochure discusses the social and financial implications of the issue and includes relevant facts and figures.

Infertility: The Emotional Roller Coaster, by Sally Cook and Ruth Streeter and edited by Linda D. Applegarth, Ed.D., discusses the various emotional "crises" that a couple may experience when one or both are infertile. Such topics as coping with family and friends and how men and women react differently to the cycles of infertility are included.

Insights into Infertility, by Catherine H. Garner, R.N.C., M.S.N., Barbara Eck Menning, R.N., and Anne Colston Wentz, M.D., a booklet that gives a comprehensive overview of male and female infertility, treatments available, and other suggested readings and resources. It also includes a glossary with over 250 basic infertility terms.

Male Infertility, by Larry I. Lipshultz, M.D., provides the patient with information on diagnosis and treatment, including commonly asked questions.

The Over 35 Infertile Patient: Special Issues, a booklet that addresses the needs of the ever-growing populations of infertile couples. It is this group who are encouraged to start their initial workup after only six months of trying to achieve a pregnancy. They often face multiple factors contributing to their infertility, and unfortunately, experience a higher miscarriage rate.

Pathways to Parenthood, by Catherine H. Garner, R.N.C., M.S.N., M.A., and Grant W. Patton, Jr., M.D., a booklet written to assist couples who are thinking of having a child. It discusses how to enhance their overall health, how conception occurs, and when and why to be concerned if pregnancy does not happen.

INSURANCE

See Health Insurance.

INTERSTITIAL CYSTITIS (IC)

See also Urinary Problems.

Interstitial cystitis is an inflammation of the bladder wall, the causes and cures of which are unknown. It can affect a person of any age. Its symptoms include

- Frequency, which can be as much as 60 times a day
- Urgency, the sensation of having to urinate immediately
- Pain, which can be abdominal, urethral, and genital

INTERSTITIAL CYSTITIS ASSOCIATION OF AMERICA, INC. *1-619-543-8954*
P.O. Box 151323
San Diego, CA 92175

Purpose The Association seeks to support IC victims and their families, educate both health care professionals and the general public, and generate funding for research. It does not make referrals to physicians but does offer telephone support by providing names and numbers of members willing to take calls.

Publications

Do You Have IC? a 1-page checklist of IC symptoms.

The Interstitial Cystitis Association, a brochure about the condition—who gets it, treatment options.

Brochure about other lower urinary tract disorders.

INTESTINAL DISEASES

See National Foundation for Ileitis and Colitis and Crohn's Disease and Colitis Foundation, pages 79, 175.

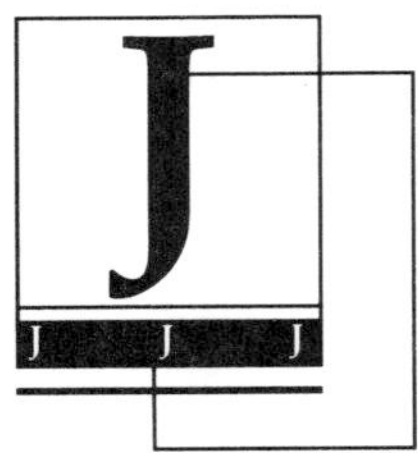

JOSEPH'S DISEASE

Machado-Joseph's is an inherited degenerative disease that affects the spine and brain.

NATIONAL INSTITUTE OF NEUROLOGICAL DISORDERS AND STROKE (NINDS) *1-301-496-5751*
Building 31, Room 8A06
Bethesda, MD 20892

Publication
Joseph's Disease, NIH Pub. No. 85-2716.

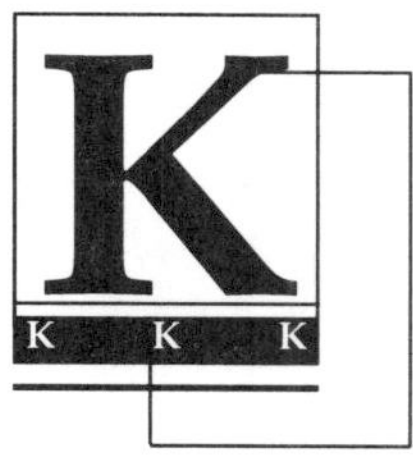

Kidney

See also Polycystic Kidney Disease.

The kidneys are situated close to the spine in the upper part of the abdomen. The chief function of the kidney is to clear certain toxins and waste compounds, together with excess fluid, from the blood. The basic functional unit of the kidney is called the nephron, which contains glomeruli, small tufts of tiny blood vessels. The glomeruli excrete fluid and waste compounds from the blood into the tubules of the kidney. Urine is formed by the glomerulus and then passes through a system of ducts to the bladder before being excreted. Because of the kidney's job in filtering chemicals, it is not surprising that many drugs and chemicals can cause kidney damage. Infections also take their toll. Kidney and urinary tract diseases affect an estimated 20 million Americans and directly cause more than 95,000 deaths each year. To help protect your kidneys from harm or to deal with kidney problems once they have occurred, obtain information from the following.

American Association of Kidney Patients — *1-813-251-0725*
111 S. Parker Street, Suite 405 — *1-800-749-2257*
Tampa, FL 33612 — *Fax 1-813-254-3270*

Purpose This voluntary, patient organization, has for more than 20 years been dedicated to helping renal patients and their families deal with the physical and emotional impact of kidney disease. The programs offered by AAKP inform and inspire patients and their families to understand better their condition, adjust more readily to their circumstances, and assume more normal, productive lives in their community.

Publications

ADA Brochure, describes the impact of the Americans with Disabilities Act on renal patients.

Blood Chemistry Values, a sheet describing what levels mean in the most often done tests.

BULLETIN, a newspaper published quarterly.

NA-K Counter-Potassium/Salt Levels for Various Foods, a pamphlet.

RENALIFE, a magazine published twice a year.

AMERICAN KIDNEY FUND *1-301-881-3052*
6110 Executive Blvd., Suite 1010 *1-800-638-8299*
Rockville, MD 20852

Purpose The Fund is a national voluntary health organization that provides direct financial assistance, comprehensive educational programs, research grants, and community service projects for the benefit of kidney patients.

Publications

One copy of the following publications are available free:

American Kidney Fund Helps When Nobody Else Will, a brochure on the services offered by the Fund. Also available in Spanish.

Application for Financial Assistance.

Bumper stickers—*Kidney Donors Save Lives.*

Children and Kidney Disease, a 17-page booklet explaining the conditions that can affect a child's kidneys and gives the warning signs.

Diabetes and the Kidneys, a 21-page booklet that provides a guide to dealing with diabetes and the kidneys and includes information about kidney transplants. Also available in large print.

The Dialysis Patient: An Informative Guide for the Dentist, a 9-page booklet that explains the special care dialysis patients need when undergoing dental treatments.

Diet Guide for the CAPD Patient.

Diet Guide for CAPD, a brochure for continuous ambulatory peritoneal dialysis patients, it offers information on calories, sodium, potassium, fluids, vitamins, and fiber. Also available in Spanish.

Diet Guide for the Hemodialysis Patient, a brochure on the nutrient needs of a patient undergoing hemodialysis. Also available in Spanish.

Directory of Public/Professional Educational Materials.

Facts About Kidney Diseases and Their Treatment, a 14-page booklet about causes and symptoms of kidney disease.

Facts About Kidney Stones, a brochure that explains kidney stones that affect from 200,000 to 1.4 million people in the United States. These figures include persons afflicted with "silent stones," as explained in the brochure.

Give a Kidney—A Guide For Organ Donation, explains the Uniform Anatomical Gift Act and includes a uniform donor card. Also available in Spanish.

High Blood Pressure and Its Effects on the Kidneys—I Am Joe's Kidney, a booklet that describes how untreated hypertension will cause damage to kidneys and other organs.

The Kid, a 17-page booklet that explains the workings of the kidneys in an entertaining way for children.

Kidney Disease: A Guide for Patients and Their Families, a 26-page booklet that describes the various forms of kidney disease, treatments, resources available, publications, and a chart for keeping track of medications. Also available in Spanish.

Kidneys for Kids, a 28-page booklet written for children who have kidney disease. It explains transplants and medications in easy-to-understand language.

The Nephrology Letter, a newsletter.

Newsletter for Health Professionals.

Organ donor cards, free.

Taking Care of Yourself: An Introduction to Peritoneal Dialysis.

Understanding Nephrotic Syndrome, a 12-page booklet that explains the kidney disease that allows protein which is normally in the blood to leak into the urine. It describes treatments and diet.

NATIONAL INSTITUTE OF DIABETES AND DIGESTIVE AND KIDNEY DISEASES *1-301-499-3583*
Building 31, Room 9A04
Bethesday, MD 20892

Publications

Prevention and Treatment of Kidney Stones, NIH Pub. No. 83-2495

Extracorporeal Shock-Wave Lithotripsy. A Treatment for Kidney Stones, NIH Pub. No. 88-859.

NATIONAL KIDNEY FOUNDATION *1-800-622-9010*
30 East 33rd St.
New York, NY 10016

Purpose The National Kidney Foundation is a voluntary health agency seeking the total answer to diseases of the kidney and urinary tract prevention, treatment, and cure. The Foundation's many-faceted program brings help and hope to many Americans who suffer from kidney and urinary tract disease through research, patient services, a nationwide organ donor program, professional education, and public information.

Publications

Blood Pressure and Your Kidneys, a brochure explaining what high blood pressure is, how high blood pressure is diagnosed and treated, who is at risk for developing high blood pressure, and how high blood pressure and kidney disease are interrelated. Additional information includes drugs that are used to treat high blood pressure and their side effects.

Coping Effectively: A Guide for Patients and Their Families, a 20-page booklet providing information on many topics of concern to patients and families, including what types of treatments are available, how treatments are paid for, whether dialysis patients should return to work, and other activities such as exercise, whether women on dialysis can have children, and much more.

Drug Abuse Can Damage Your Kidneys, a brochure aimed at informing young people about how alcohol and drugs such as cocaine, heroin, and amphetamines can affect their kidneys.

Patient Services: Dedicated to Quality of Life, a brochure providing information on the wide variety of patient and community services offered by the National Kidney Foundation through its local affiliates. Among the services described are education programs, support groups, financial assistance, social and recreational programs, patient advocacy, resource development, rehabilitation programs, transportation programs, and information and referral services.

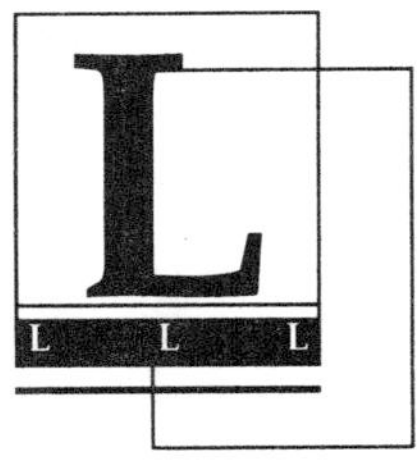

LABORATORY TOPICS

AMERICAN SOCIETY OF CLINICAL PATHOLOGISTS *1-312-738-1336*
2100 West Harrison St.
Chicago, IL 60612-3798

Purpose A not-for-profit medical society organized for educational, scientific, and charitable purposes, the ASCP's mission is to promote public health and safety. Founded in 1922, the Society is the largest pathology organization in the world. Its members consist of about 11,000 pathologists and other physicians and more than 40,000 laboratory professionals, including doctoral-level laboratory scientists, medical technologists, cytotechnologists, histotechnologists, and medical laboratory technicians. These efforts include the appropriate application of pathology and laboratory medicine and serving as the national resource to enhance the quality of pathology and laboratory medicine. The ASCP develops comprehensive educational programs and materials. No referrals are made to physicians.

Publications
A wide range, including career information for aspiring pathologists and medical laboratory professionals and patient education materials, with many on laboratory topics such as *pap smears* and such conditions as *cancer, diabetes, Lyme disease,* and *thyroid.* The ASC asks that you phone first for information on the subject of interest.

LEARNING DISABILITIES

See also Attention Deficit Disorders *and* Dyslexia.

If your child is having trouble learning to speak, read, or write relative to other children of the same age, he or she may just be a little slow to develop these skills and will eventually catch up, or your child may have a learning problem. The cause may be as simple as needed eyeglasses or a hearing aid or may be more complicated. Early and accurate diagnosis and therapy are vital if a learning disability does exist.

LEARNING DISABILITIES ASSOCIATION OF AMERICA *1-412-341-1515*
4156 Library Road
Pittsburgh, PA 15234

Purpose The Association is a national information and referral service having local chapters throughout the country. Information for parents, professionals, and adults with learning disabilities.

Publications

A Guide to Section 504, a publication explaining the section of the Rehabilitation Act of 1973 that applies to persons with disabilities.

Learning Disabilities—What Is It? a brochure describing symptoms with a checklist.

Taking the First Step to Solve Learning Disabilities, a brochure discussing goals, legislation, and other goals of the organization.

NATIONAL CENTER FOR LEARNING DISABILITIES (NCLD) *1-212-687-7211*
99 Park Avenue
New York, NY 10016

Purpose Between 10 and 15 percent of the U.S. population has some form of learning disabilities. The National Center for Learning Disabilities helps those affected with this "hidden handicap" live self-sufficient, productive, and fulfilling lives. NCLD provides information and referrals and educational programs and projects. It raises public awareness and understanding and advocates legislation. It will refer through a national information service.

Publication

Resourceful Parents, a list of recommended books, newsletters, and periodicals about LDs.

LEGIONNAIRE'S DISEASE

See Infectious Diseases *and* Laboratory Topics.

LEPROSY (HANSEN'S DISEASE)

Leprosy is a chronic infectious disease caused by a bacteria, *M. Leprae*. It has a prolonged incubation period (from 1 to 30 years) and progresses slowly. An ancient, legendary scourge, it is now found mainly within Southeast Asia, Africa, and South America. Of the estimated 12 to 20 million cases, about 2,000 are in the continental United States, mostly in Texas, Louisiana, and Hawaii. The disease has also been diagnosed in California, Florida, and New York City among immigrants. It can be cured if prompt therapy is given.

ALM INTERNATIONAL *1-803-271-7040*
1 A.L.M. Way *1-800-543-3131*
Greenville, SC 29601

Purpose This organization educates the public and raises funds for cure of leprosy and for rehabilitation in 25 countries. ALM sends support to hospitals and clinics worldwide and makes referrals to ten regional outpatient contract hospitals in the United States. Calls are also often directed to ALM's medical director.

Publications
Questions People Ask About Leprosy.
Word & Deed, a quarterly newsletter.
Various other materials.

LEUKODYSTROPHY

Leukodystrophy refers to a group of disorders that affect the brain, spinal cord, and peripheral nerves. The word "leukodystrophy" derives from the Greek words *leuko,* meaning "white" and alluding to the white matter of the nervous system and *dystrophy,* meaning imperfect growth or development. The cause of leukodystrophy is an inherited problem in one specific chemical reaction necessary to maintain the myelin sheaths, the covering of nerve fibers.

UNITED LEUKODYSTROPHY FOUNDATION, INC. *1-815-895-3211*
2304 Highland Drive *1-800-728-5483*
Sycamore, IL 60178

Purpose A nonprofit, voluntary health organization, it provides leukodystrophy patients and their families with information about leukodystrophy and assists them in identifying sources of medical care, social services, and genetic counseling. Will refer to physicians and self-help groups.

LIBRARIES, MEDICAL

See Medical Libraries.

LIPID STORAGE DISEASE

Abnormal levels of blood or tissue fats resulting from metabolic disorders that may be inborn or due to hormonal disorders, specific organ failure, or external causes.

NATIONAL INSTITUTE OF NEUROLOGICAL DISORDERS AND STROKE (NINDS) *1-301-496-5751*
Building 31, Room 8A06
Bethesda, MD 20892

Publication
Lipid Storage Disease, NIH Pub. No. 84-2628.

LIVER

The liver is the largest single internal organ. It fills the upper right-hand part of the abdomen behind the lower ribs. The liver has a vital role in regulating the composition of the blood and also plays a large part in many other body processes. One function of the liver is to make bile, a green fluid that helps breakdown fat and another is to detoxify chemicals. Liver diseases include viral infections such as hepatitis and cirrhosis. Drug reactions can also harm the liver.

AMERICAN LIVER FOUNDATION *1-800-223-0179*
1425 Pompton Avenue
Cedar Grove, NJ 07009

Purpose The American Liver Foundation is the only national health organization dedicated to finding cures for liver disease by supporting research, providing professional and public educational programs, and promoting liver wellness and awareness. The Foundation has chapters nationwide that provide support and education for patients struggling with liver disease and their families. It will provide referrals to physicians specializing in liver problems.

Publications
Provides a list of publications and videocassettes for sale.

LOWE'S SYNDROME

The disease occurs in male infants and inheritance is consistent with a sex linked recessive pattern. The neurological symptoms include severe mental retardation, convulsions, flabby muscles, cataracts, glaucoma, undescended testicles and rickets. The fundamental defect is unknown and there is no specific treatment.

LOWE'S SYNDROME ASSOCIATION (LSA) *1-317-743-3634*
222 Lincoln St.
West Lafayette, IN 47906

Purpose A nonprofit organization, LSA seeks to foster communication among families of people with Lowe's syndrome, to provide medical and educational information, and to encourage research into the cause and prevention of the disease. Interested in Lowe's syndrome, oculocerebrorenal syndrome, genetic diseases, multiply handicapped children, visual impairment and blindness, kidney disease, mental retardation, genetic research and counseling, X-linked conditions, and metabolism, the Association answers inquiries; conducts seminars, workshops, and national meetings (irregular); distributes publications; and makes referrals to other sources of information. Services are primarily for members, but others will be assisted.

Publications

Care Today—Cure Tomorrow, basic informational brochure and membership form for the LSA.

Living With Lowe's Syndrome: A Guide for Families, Friends, and Professionals, a booklet that provides medical and developmental information about Lowe's syndrome. Includes genetics, research, and effect on the family.

LUNGS

LUNGLINE® *1-800-222-LUNG*
1-303-355-LUNG (in Denver)

A free information service staffed by specially trained National Jewish Center nurses to provide information about breathing difficulties, and allergic, occupation, or immune system diseases.

Publications

BROCHURES

Being Close (sex and respiratory illness).

Black Lung Disease.

Healthy Breathing

Juvenile Rheumatoid Arthritis.

Management of Chronic Respiratory Disease.

Nocturnal Asthma, an 8-page brochure that explains how respiratory diseases, particularly asthma, have the potential to change greatly during sleep.

Understanding Allergy, brochure describing allergy in general, diagnosis, and treatments available.

Understanding Asthma, a brochure defining asthma and describing how to live with the condition.

Understanding Emphysema, a brochure explaining the symptoms and physiology of the crippling lung condition that affects more than 2.4 million Americans and that kills 13,000 of them every year.

Understanding Immunology.

Your Child and Asthma, a 20-page brochure that discusses in addition to symptoms and treatment, the costs in emotion and money.

MEDICAL FACT SHEETS

Alpha-l Antitrypsin Deficiency (inherited emphysema).
Allergic and Nonallergic Rhinitis (hayfever).
Allergy Testing.
Allergy to Animals and Pets.
Antibiotics and Asthma.
Asthma and Pregnancy.
Asthma Triggers.
Atypical Mycobacteria.
Atrovent.
Beryllium Disease.
Bronchiectasis.
Chronic Bronchitis.
Chest Assessment.
Cleaning Humidifiers/Vaporizers.
Cleaning Nebulizers.
Cromolyn.
Eczema/Atopic Dermatitis.
Efficacy Data.
Environmental Control.
Emphysema.
Exercise and Asthma.
Interstitial Lung Disease.
Immunotherapy.
Infections in Children.
Management of COPD.
Metabisulfites.
Metered Dose Inhalers.
Moving.
New Drugs for Asthma.
Over-the-Counter Asthma Medications.
Parenting Asthmatic Children.
Pneumonia.
Pride Program.
Pulmonary Rehabilitation.
Passive Smoking.
Reading List—Emphysema.
Reading List—Asthma.
Sarcoidosis.

Sinusitis and Asthma.
Systemic Lupus Erythematosus.
Sleep Apnea.
Smoking Literature.
Spirometry.
Steroids.
Steroids at a Glance.
Theophylline Questions and Answers.
Time Management/Pacing.
Teacher's Memo.
Tuberculosis.

NATIONAL HEART, LUNG, AND BLOOD INSTITUTE *1-301-496-4236*
Building 31, Room 4A21
Bethesda, MD 20892

Publications
Chronic Obstructive Pulmonary Disease, NIH Pub. No. 86-2020.
Do I Have a Chronic Cough? NIH Pub. No. 89-559.
Eat Right to Facts About Asthma, NIH Pub. No. 90-2339.

NATIONAL INSTITUTES OF HEALTH (NIH) *1-301-496-2563*
Office of Clinical Center Communications
Building 10, Room 1C255
Bethesda, MD 20892

Publication
The Lungs.

NATIONAL JEWISH CENTER FOR IMMUNOLOGY AND RESPIRATORY MEDICINE *1-303-388-4461*
1400 Jackson St.
Denver, CO 80206

LUPUS

Systemic *Lupus erythematosus*, commonly called "lupus," is a disease of the body's immune system. Its symptoms include a butterfly rash over the nose and cheeks, weakness, fatigue, weight loss, and arthritis. As the disease advances, it may damage major organs, leading to kidney failure, strokes, seizures, or respiratory arrest. Lupus affects as many as 1 million Americans. Over 50,000 new cases are diagnosed each year.

LUPUS FOUNDATION OF AMERICA, INC. *1-301-670-9292*
4 Research Place, Suite 180 *1-800-558-0121*
Rockville, MD 20850-3226

Purpose The Foundation seeks to promote public awareness of lupus, to provide patient and physician education on lupus, to provide support and service to our nearly 100 chapters nationwide, and to support research into the causes, cure, and treatments for lupus. On the national level, the foundation offers information, publications, educational materials. On the chapter level, support groups, information, physician referral, education, and information are provided.

Publications

A list of lupus publications—including some in other languages—is available.

NATIONAL INSTITUTE OF ARTHRITIS *1-301-496-8188*
AND MUSCULOSKELETAL AND SKIN DISEASES (NIAMSD)
Building 31, Room 4C05
Bethesda, MD 20892

Publications

Disorders Update: Lupus Erythematosus Research, NIH Pub. No. 87-460.
What Black Women Should Know About Lupus, NIH Pub. No. 91-3219.

TERRI GOTTHELF LUPUS RESEARCH INSTITUTE *1-800-203-8787*
3 Duke Place
South Norwalk, CT 06854

Purpose The Terri Gotthelf Lupus Research Institute was founded and named in memory of Terri Gotthelf who lost her life to lupus at 21 years. The Institute was founded to help the millions of lupus victims in the world and to encourage, coordinate, and direct future progress in the etiology, diagnosis, and treatment of this disease. In addition to funding research, the Institute publishes materials which bring to the attention of clinicians, scientists, and the public new accomplishments in lupus research.

LYME DISEASE

Each year more and more people are discovering that a seemingly innocent tick bite can cause Lyme disease, initially a flulike illness that can lead to heart and nerve disorders, hepatitis, arthritis, and in rare cases death. Experts in laboratory medicine with the American Society of Clinical Pathologists say early diagnosis and treatment can arrest the serious long-term effects that the disease causes in about 50 to 80 percent of the untreated victims. Lyme disease is caused by *Borrelia burgdorferi* bacteria transmitted by the bite of infected ticks. These ticks require animal hosts, mainly the white-footed mouse and white-tailed deer. Up to 80 percent of the people with Lyme disease develop a characteristic bull's-eye rash.

AMERICAN SOCIETY OF CLINICAL PATHOLOGISTS *1-312-738-4886*
2100 W. Harrison Street *Fax 312-738-1619*
Chicago, IL 60612

Publication

Send a stamped, self-addressed, business-size envelope for

Lyme Disease: A Summer Threat (PH), describing the symptoms, laboratory tests, and treatments for the condition.

ARTHRITIS FOUNDATION *1-800-283-7833*
P.O. Box 19000
Atlanta, GA 30326

Publication

Lyme Disease, No. 4275.

LYME BORRELIOSIS FOUNDATION, INC. *1-203-871-2900*
P.O. Box 462
Tolland, CT 06084-0462

Purpose The Lyme Borreliosis Foundation, Inc. (LBF), is a nonprofit foundation formed in March, 1988 to be a coordinator for *Lyme borreliosis* (Lyme disease) and related disorders. The Foundation's services include public education, sponsoring national and regional conferences on Lyme disease, supporting research into the condition, organizing support groups, and providing medical referrals to Lyme disease victims. The LBF has also established the first nationwide Lyme Disease and Pregnancy Registry. This program will follow the progress of women who have Lyme disease during their pregnancy, make available information regarding treatment protocols, and provide testing options both during the pregnancy and after the birth to determine the presence of Lyme infection in the mother and child for a year after birth. The Foundation refers patients to Lyme knowledgeable physicians upon request.

Publication

List of publications, pamphlets, videos and slideshows for purchase.

LYME DISEASE RESOURCE NETWORK — *1-708-215-3819*
455 Knightbridge Parkway — *1-800-215-0288*
Lincolnshire, IL 60069

Purpose The Network provides information about Lyme disease and its treatments. It will provide names of a specialist in the treatment of Lyme disease in your area.

NATIONAL INSTITUTES OF HEALTH (NIH) — *1-301-496-2563*
Office of Clinical Center Communications
Building 10, Room 1C255
Bethesda, MD 20892

Publication
Lyme Disease, a video that can be borrowed.

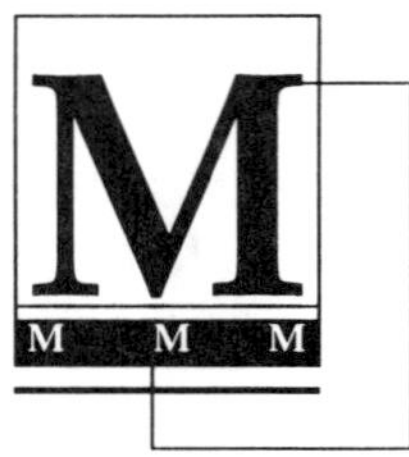

Macular Disease

The macula, the area of the back of the eye near the optic nerve, is that part of the eye that distinguishes fine detail at the center of the field of vision. Its degeneration is the leading cause of dimming vision in the elderly. A blood deficiency that sometimes occurs with age may cause macula degeneration. It can be a slow or sudden but painless loss of central vision. No medical therapy is effective. Vision can sometimes be improved, however, by magnifying eyeglasses.

Association for Macular Diseases *1-212-605-3719*
210 E. 64th St.
New York, NY 10021

Purpose The Association's aim is to bring hope, comfort, and practical suggestions to persons suffering from macular diseases and to establish and fund an eye bank exclusively devoted to research as to the causes and possible cures for macular diseases. The Association helps to develop local support groups, sponsors educational seminars, and offers an information line and referral to physicians specializing in the problem.

Publications
A brochure about the association.
A quarterly newsletter.

Marfan's Syndrome

Marfan's syndrome involves degeneration of connective tissue, especially in the skeleton, lungs, eyes, heart, and blood vessels. It is a genetic disorder. Marfan symptoms include loose joints, curvature of the spine, nearsightedness, and heart defects.

National Center for Research Resources *1-301-496-5545*
Westwood Building, Room 857
Bethesda, MD 20892

Publication

Advances in Treatment of Marfan's Syndrome.

NATIONAL MARFAN FOUNDATION *1-516-883-8712*
382 Main Street *1-800-8-MARFAN*
Port Washington, NY 11050

Purpose Disseminates accurate and timely information about the Marfan syndrome to patients, family members, and physicians. Provides a means for patients and relatives to share experiences, support one another, and improve their medical care and to foster research. Refers to chapters and support groups.

Publications

The Marfan Syndrome: A Booklet for Teachers

The Marfan Syndrome: Physical Activity Guidelines for Coaches, Physical Educators and Physicians.

MASSAGE THERAPY

Massage is an ancient method of easing sore muscles and tense emotions. A back or neck rub is a common way for a friend or family member to sooth someone's painfully tense muscles. Physiotherapists and skilled masseurs and masseuses use massage to soften muscles in spasm and to stretch muscles and joints to allow the recipient of their hands on therapy to gain greater freedom for exercise, work, and daily activity.

AMERICAN MASSAGE THERAPY ASSOCIATION *1-312-761-2682*
1130 W. North Shore Ave.
Chicago, IL 60626

Purpose Founded in 1943, AMTA is the oldest and largest national organization representing the interests of the massage therapy profession. AMTA is dedicated to the advancement of the art, science, and practice of massage therapy in a caring, professional, and ethical manner. AMTA's membership of more than 13,700 represents a wide variety of massage therapy and bodywork disciplines. The organization maintains a national consumer information and referral service.

Publications

A Guide to Massage Therapy in America.

Publication list of booklets and videotapes.

MASTECTOMY

See Breast Cancer.

MEDICAL DEVICES

The geniuses of American medicine have provided mechanical devices and artificial organs to make up for what is missing or lost in the body. Sometimes, like a TV or a car, the gizmo does not work properly.

DEVICE EXPERIENCE NETWORK *1-800-638-6725*
Division of Product Surveillance
Office of Compliance and Surveillance
Center for Devices and Radiological Health (FDA)
FDA HFZ-343
8757 Georgia Ave.
Silver Spring, MD 20910

MEDICAL EMERGENCIES

See Emergencies.

MEDICAL LIBRARIES

A source of information for any ailment that afflicts humans can be found in most medical libraries. Librarians are almost always very cooperative in providing information to public inquiries.

MEDICAL AND CHIRUGICAL FACULTY OF THE STATE OF MARYLAND LIBRARY *1-800-492-1056 (Maryland only)*
1211 Cathedral St.
Baltimore, MD 21201

NATIONAL LIBRARY OF MEDICINE *1-800-638-8480*
8600 Rockville Pike
Bethesda, MD 20894

MEDICATIONS

Each year Americans take 1.6 billion prescriptions. Improper use of prescription medicines costs the economy between $10 and $15 billion per year. American businesses lose about 20 million work days due to incorrect use of medicines prescribed for heart and circulatory diseases alone. Ninety six percent of patients don't ask any questions about their prescriptions. As for non-prescription drugs, there are 600,000 products available for self-medication

COUNCIL ON FAMILY HEALTH *1-212-598-3617*
225 Park Avenue South, Suite 1700
New York, NY 10003

Purpose The Council on Family Health, a nonprofit organization dedicated to educating consumers on the proper use of medicines, provides educational materials.

Publications

Medicines and You: A Guide for Older Americans
Nonprescription Medicines: A Consumer's Dictionary of Terms. Also available in Spanish.

FOOD AND DRUG ADMINISTRATION (FDA) *1-301-443-3170*
HFE-88
Public and Professional Affairs Dept.
5600 Fishers Lane
Rockville, MD 20857

Publication

How to Take Your Medicine: Penicillins (Spanish version, FDA 91-3184S), reprint of *FDA Consumer* article.

NATIONAL INFORMATION CENTER FOR ORPHAN DRUGS & RARE DISEASES *1-800-336-4797*
P.O. Box 1133
Washington, DC 20013

NATIONAL INSTITUTE OF GENERAL MEDICAL SCIENCES (NIGMS) *1-301-496-7301*
Office of Research Reports
Building 31, Room 4A52
Bethesda, MD 20892

Publication

Medicines and You, NIH Pub. No. 81-2140. Your age, your genes, and your diet can all affect the way medicines work in your body. This booklet describes what medical researchers are learning about the biological individuality of each human being and how this individuality affects the nature of each person's responses to medicines and other chemicals.

MEDICINE (INTERNAL)

Internal medicine is concerned with the medical, rather than the surgical or obstetrical, diagnosis and therapy of diseases of adults. Physicians in this specialty are called internists. There are several subspecialties within internal medicine in which the physician has a particular training in diagnosis and treatment. These include cardiology, gastroenterology, and hematology.

AMERICAN COLLEGE OF PHYSICIANS *1-215-351-2400*
Public Education
Independence Mall West
6th Street at Race
Philadelphia, PA 19106-1572

Purpose The American College of Physicians, the nation's largest medical specialty society, works to uphold health care standards through activities in continuing education, health policy analysis, quality assurance, and medical technology assessment. Its membership includes more than 70,000 primary care physicians and specialists in the various branches of internal medicine. Disciplines within or related to internal medicine include cardiology, gastroenterology, nephrology, endocrinology, hematology, dermatology, allergy and immunology, psychiatry, critical care medicine, geriatrics, and occupational medicine.

Publications

ACP Health Library, a bimonthly patient education series with materials for patients and physicians. The pamphlets help clarify health issues for patients. Recent topics include cholesterol, screening for colorectal cancer, the skin and ultraviolet light, osteoporosis, adult immunization, and smoking cessation.

MEMORY

Intelligence is the capacity to learn. Learning is based on the acquisition of new knowledge about the environment. Memory is its retention. The storage of data in our brains requires three basic things:

1. *Registration*. Our brain must receive the information from our senses.
2. *Consolidation*. The information has to be stored either short term or long term.
3. *Retrieval*. We have to be able to call up that information when we want it.

NEW JERSEY NEUROLOGICAL INSTITUTE® 1-201-992-3300
MEMORY ENHANCEMENT CLINIC®
22 Old Short Hills Road
Livingston, NJ 07039

Purpose Founded in 1976, New Jersey Neurological Institute® is a multidisciplinary group of professionals dedicated to aiding individuals who suffer from acute and chronic neurological problems. The Memory Enhancement Clinic® assesses and treats memory problems with state-of-the-art techniques and equipment.

Publications
Send a stamped, self-addressed, business-size envelope for
New Jersey Neurological's Brief Memory Test.
Ten Ways to Preserve Your Memory.

MENOPAUSE

Menopause is the time in a woman's life when the ovaries produce decreasing levels of hormones and menstrual periods have ceased for at least one year.

THE SUPERINTENDENT OF DOCUMENTS
USGPO
Washington, D.C. 20402

Publication
The Menopause Time of Life, NIH Pub. No. 86-2461.

MENTAL HEALTH

Mental illnesses include a variety of relatively severe mental disorders that interfere significantly with people's abilities to live and work. More hospital beds are occupied by people with serious mental illnesses than by any other illness. There are many exciting research advances in both diagnosis and treatment.

AMERICAN ASSOCIATION FOR MUSIC THERAPY (AAMT) 215-265-4006
P.O. Box 80012
Valley Forge, PA 19484

Purpose The Association is dedicated to establishing standards of professional competence, implementing those standards through certification of individuals and approval of university curricula, promoting and disseminating research through professional publications, fostering community awareness and public education in regard to the goals and applications of music therapy, developing employment opportunities, developing continuing education curricula reflective of new trends in the field, and improving the quality of life through the use of music in therapy.

Publications
AAMT brochure contains information regarding membership, publications, education, certification, and competencies.

AMERICAN PSYCHIATRIC ASSOCIATION *1-202-682-6220*
Division of Public Affairs/Code P-H
1400 K Street, N.W.
Washington, D.C. 20005

Purpose The Division of Public Affairs conducts a nationwide mental illnesses awareness campaign aimed at improving public understanding of mental illnesses and psychiatric treatment. Responds to public inquiries; refers to local psychiatric societies.

Publications
Anxiety.
Childhood Disorders.
Choosing a Psychiatrist.
Depression.
Let's Talk About Mental Illnesses, a catalog listing print and audiovisual materials.
Let's Talk Facts About Mental Illness, 14-title series of information pamphlets on various mental illnesses.
Mental Health of the Elderly.
Mental Illnesses: There Are a Lot of Troubled People.
Obsessive-Compulsive Disorder.
Panic Disorders.
Post-Traumatic Stress Disorder.
Schizophrenia.
Substance Abuse.
Teen Suicide.

AMERICAN PSYCHOLOGICAL ASSOCIATION (APA) *1-202-955-7710*
750 First St., N.E. *1-800-296-0272*
Washington, D.C. 20002 *Fax 1-202-331-0437*

Purpose The APA is the major organization representing psychology in the United States. Established in 1892, it has various divisions which collectively advance psychology as a science, profession, and means of promoting human welfare. More than 70,000 members belong and cover 50 areas of psychology. The APA will refer to therapists in your area but not to a self-help group.

Publications

Among the free brochures are

AIDS.
Alcoholism.
Black Males in America.
Careers in Psychology.
Childhood Depression: Youth Suicide.
Children and Drugs.
Children and T.V.: Using T.V. Sensibly.
Choosing a Psychotherapist.
Compulsive Gambling.
Depression: What You Need to Know.
Does Adoption Mean Different?
Drugs—Use, Misuse, Abuse: Guidance for Families.
Finding the Right Psychotherapist.
Good Mental Health.
If Sex Enters into the Therapy Relationship.
The Mind/Body Connection.
One-Parent Families.
Preventing Armageddon.
Psychology and You.
The Psychotherapies Today.
The Retarded Child Gets Ready for School.
Sexual Behavior and Aids.
Sports Psychology.
Stepfamilies—A Growing Reality.
Teaching Your Children Self-discipline.
To Combat and Prevent Child Abuse and Neglect.
Understanding and Dealing with Alcoholism.
Understanding Stress.
The Value of Psychotherapy.
Violence on TV.
What You Should Know About Drug Abuse.
When the Trigger Pulls the Finger.
When Children Are Unwanted.
When You Need Child Day Care.

CULT AWARENESS NETWORK (CAN) *1-312-267-7777*
2421 W. Pratt Blvd., Suite 1173
Chicago, IL 60645

Purpose CAN is a national nonprofit organization founded to educate the public about the harmful effects of mind control used by destructive cults. CAN confines its concerns to unethical or illegal practices and does not judge doctrine or beliefs. It offers direct assistance to victims through FOCUS (a network for ex-members to share their experiences), special seminars, and programs. Assistance is given to victims' families through volunteer chapters across the country. CAN responds to inquiries from the public, providing free literature. CAN provides educational programs to alert educators, clergy, and mental health professionals on how to recognize and help cult victims. CAN co-sponsors the International Cult Education Project (ICEP) in conjunction with American Family Foundation to work with colleges, schools, churches, and synagogues.

Publications
CAN: Cult Awareness Network, a brochure about the organization.
Order form for books and booklets available for sale from the Network.

MENTAL ILLNESS FOUNDATION — *1-212-629-0755*
7 Penn Plaza, Suite 222
New York, NY 10001

Purpose The Foundation gives grants for medical research, residencies, and rehabilitation facilities and offers programs for the seriously mentally ill.

Publications
Directories of services for the seriously mentally ill and their families in the boroughs of New York City, and Westchester and Suffolk counties of New York.

NATIONAL ALLIANCE FOR THE MENTALLY ILL (NAMI) — *1-703-524-7600*
2101 Wilson Blvd., Suite 302 — *Fax 1-703-524-9094*
Arlington, VA 22201

Purpose A self-help organization with over 1,000 local affiliates throughout the United States whose members include 140,000 relatives and friends of people with mental illnesses and those people themselves. NAMI emphasizes mutual support, public education, research, and advocacy to improve the lives of people with serious mental illnesses.

NATIONAL MENTAL HEALTH ASSOCIATION (NMHA) — *1-703-684-7722*
1021 Prince St. — *1-800-969-NMHA*
Alexandria, VA 22314-2971 — *Fax 703-684-5968*

Purpose The Association promotes advocacy and education about mental health and has many educational materials on mental health and mental illness; it will refer to self-help groups only.

Publications
FOCUS, NMHA's official newsletter.

Prevention Update.
Publications list with pamphlets, videotapes, federal program summaries, policy resources, and general information. Some pamphlets are about 10 to 35 cents each.

NATIONAL INSTITUTE OF AGING (NIA) *1-301-496-1752*
Public Inquiries
Federal Building, Room 6C12
Bethesda, MD 20892

Publication

Safe Use of Tranquilizers.

NATIONAL INSTITUTE OF MENTAL HEALTH (NIMH) *1-301-443-2403*
Information Resources and Inquiries Branch
Office of Scientific Information, Room 15C
5900 Fishers Lane, Room 15-105
Rockville, MD 20857

Publications

The NIMH asks that you request only ten publications.

AIDS

When Someone Close Has AIDS: Acquired Immunodeficiency Syndrome, ADM 89-1515, 15 pages.

ALZHEIMER'S DISEASE

There Were Times, Dear . . . Living with Alzheimer's Disease, OM 87-4023, 21 pages.
Useful Information on Alzheimer's Disease, ADM 90-1696, 24 pages.

ATTITUDES

Affirmative Action to Employ Mentally Restored People, ADM 81-1073, 18 pages.
Eight Questions Employers Ask About Hiring the Mentally Restored, ADM 81-1072, 17 pages.
Plain Talk About the Stigma of Mental Illness, ADM 90-1470, 4 pages.
The 14 Worst Myths About Recovered Mental Patients, ADM 89-1391, 16 pages.

CHILD AND FAMILY

Helping the Hyperactive Child. Caring About Kids Series, ADM 85-561, 9 pages.
Importance of Play. Caring About Kids Series, ADM 81-0969, 16 pages.

Learning While Growing: Cognitive Development. Caring About Kids Series, ADM 81-1017, 14 pages.
Plain Talk About Adolescence, ADM 85-1065, 2 pages.
Pre-Term Babies. Caring About Kids Series, ADM 80-0972, 15 pages.
Stimulating Baby Senses. Caring About Kids Series, ADM 77-0481, 10 pages.
When Parents Divorce. Caring About Kids Series, ADM 8l-1120, 22 pages.

DEPRESSION

Beating Depression: New Treatments Bring Success, reprinted from *U.S. News and World Report*, March 5 1990, OM 00-4053, 8 pages.
Bipolar Disorder: Manic. Depressive Illness, ADM 90-1609, 6 pages.
D/ART Fact Sheet, ADM 90-1680, 2 pages.
Depression: It's a Disease and It Can Be Treated, reprinted from *Discover*, Vol. 7, No. 5, May 1986, OM 00-4028, 10 pages.
Depressive Illnesses: Treatments Bring New Hope, ADM 89-1491, 28 pages.
Helpful Facts About Depressive Disorders, ADM 89-1536, 8 pages.
Helping the Depressed Person Get Treatment, ADM 90-1675, 23 pages.
If You're over 65 and Feeling Depressed . . . Treatment Brings New Hope, ADM 90-1653, 12 pages.
Let's Talk About Depression, ADM 91-1695, 2 pages, prepared especially for young blacks.
Plain Talk About Depression, ADM 90-1639, 4 pages.
What to do When a Friend is Depressed: A Guide For Teenagers, OM 00-4036, 8 pages.

GENERAL MENTAL HEALTH

A Consumer's Guide to Mental Health Services, ADM 87-0214, 28 pages.
Homeless Mentally Ill: Service Needs of the Population, ADM 88-1598, 10 pages.
Homeless Mentally Ill: Service Needs of the Population from the National Institute of Health, ADM 87-1520, 26 pages.
Obsessive-Compulsive Disorder: Useful Information from the NIMH, ADM 90-1597, 8 pages.
Plain Talk About Aging, ADM 85-1266, 4 pages.
Plain Talk About Handling Stress, ADM 87-0502, 2 pages.
Plain Talk About Mutual Help Groups, ADM 89-1138, 6 pages.
Plain Talk About Physical Fitness and Mental Health, ADM 84-1364, 3 pages.
Plain Talk About the Art of Relaxation, ADM 85-0632, 2 pages.
Plain Talk About Wife Abuse, ADM 85-1265, 3 pages.
Schizophrenia: Question and Answers, ADM 90-1457, 25 pages.
Useful Information on . . . Anorexia Nervosa & Bulimia, ADM 87-1514, 15 pages.
Useful Information on . . . Medications for Mental Illness, ADM 87-1509, 27 pages.
Useful Information on Paranoia, ADM-89-1495, 10 pages.
Useful Information on . . . Sleep Disorders, ADM 87-1541, 36 pages.

You Are Not Alone: Facts About Mental Health and Mental Illness, ADM 90-1178, 11 pages.

SPANISH LANGUAGE PUBLICATIONS

Charla Franca Como Tratar al Nino Enojado (Plain Talk About Dealing with the Angry Child), SP 80-0781, 4 pages.

Cuando un Amigo Tiene el S.I.D.A. (When Someone Close Has AIDS), SP 90-1515, 14 pages.

D/ART. Depresion/Advertencia, Reconocimiento, Tratamiento. Folleto Informativo (D/ART Information Flyer), OM 00-4033, 2 pages.

Datos Utiles Sobre Enfermedades Depresivas, (Helpful Facts About Depressive Disorders), SP 90-1702, 7 pages.

Depresion: Lo Que Usted Necesita Saber (Depression: What You Need to Know), SP 87-1543, 13 pages.

Esquizofrenia Preguntas y Respuestas (Schizophrenia: Questions and Answers), SP 91-1457, 28 pages.

No Estas Solo: Datos Acerca de Salud Mental y Enfermedades (You Are Not Alone: Facts About Mental Health and Mental Illness), SP 90-1178, 28 pages.

Platica Franca Sobre La Tension (Plain Talk About Stress), SP 91-0502, 4 pages.

Una Guia Sobre Servicios De Salud Mental Para Los Consumidores (Consumers Guide to Mental Health Services), SP 90-0214, 24 pages.

The NIMH maintains a collection of videotapes. If you want to order audiovisual materials, include in your order a blank videotape cassette with enough minutes on it to tape the materials you request. The NIMH Technical Services will tape the requested materials and return your videocassette to you.

Orders should be sent to

The National Institute of Mental Health
Technical Services Branch
5100 Fishers Lane, Room 14-105
Rockville, MD 20857

Just Like You and Me, 32 minutes. This video, produced in cooperation with the National Restaurant Association, features former mental patients who have made a successful transition from hospitalization back into the community and, through the Transitional Employment Program (TEP), have returned to the work force.

Making the Numbers Work for You, 35 minutes. Produced by the Division of Applied and Services Research, the videotape relates the history of the National Reporting Program for Mental Health Statistics. It points out the need for timely, accurate statistical information from each state. Such information assists the federal government in compiling figures on the needs and opportunities in promoting better mental health throughout the United States.

More than a Grant, 19 minutes. Executive Order 12677 was issued to enhance the government support of historically black colleges and universities (HBCUs). As a part of this effort to eliminate barriers that may have resulted in reduced participation by HBCUs in federally sponsored programs, NIMH has made available this tape. It describes some of the Institute's programs and should encourage HBCU faculties and students to explore ways of obtaining support for research projects in the field of mental health.

More than a Passing Acquaintance, 24 minutes. This tape tells the story of how one community support program, Way Station in Frederick, Maryland, meets the challenge in providing services and opportunities for persons who have made the successful transition from hospitalization back into the community and how some have found employment in the area.

Windows into the Brain, 19 minutes. From the NIMH Office of Scientific Information and the Division of Intramural Research, this film tells the story of three decades of scientific advances in brain imaging techniques. It includes computerized axial tomography (CAT scan), positron emission tomography (PET scan), and magnetic resonance imaging (MRI). This tape has received favorable comments from both adult audiences and junior high science students.

SEVENTH-DAY ADVENTIST COMMUNITY HEALTH SERVICES *1-516-627-2210*
P.O. Box 1029
Manhasset, NY 11030

Publication

Power to Cope, mental, physical, and spiritual guidelines in handling stress.

UNIVERSITY OF PENNSYLVANIA *1-215-898-4529*
School of Veterinary Medicine
Center for the Interaction of Animals and Society
3800 Spruce St.
Philadelphia, PA 19104

Purpose The Center studies the interaction between pets and people. One aspect is bonding and coping with grief when a pet dies. A social worker provides counseling in person or over the phone to pet owners who have lost a pet or are about to lose a pet. Also holds a bimonthly grief therapy group. Referrals are made if a social worker feels it is needed.

The Center conducts research into the interrelationships linking people to animals; disseminates knowledge about those interrelationships to veterinary students, health care professionals, and the general public; and applies this knowledge to clinical and consulting services. The Center is interested in human/animal bonding, animal behavior problems, pet bereavement counseling, and animals used in human therapy. It answers inquiries; provides advisory, reference, and copying services; and makes referrals to other sources of information. Services are free, except copying, and are available to anyone.

Publication

Bellwether, a newsletter for the school. A small donation is requested.

MENTAL RETARDATION

This appellation is now being changed to developmental disability to describe the problems of people whose mental development has been impaired. There are federal, state and private organizations that provide a wide range of services for the severely developmentally disabled.

NATIONAL INSTITUTE OF CHILD HEALTH AND HUMAN DEVELOPMENT (NICHHD) *1-301-496-5133*
Building 31, Room 2A32
Bethesda, MD 20892

Publication

Centers of Excellence: The Mental Retardation Research Centers, NIH Pub. No. 86-2882.

U.S. DEPARTMENT OF HEALTH AND HUMAN SERVICES *1-800-444-6472*
Public Health Service
Office of Minority Health Resource Center
P.O. Box 37337
Washington, D.C. 20013-7337

Purpose The U.S. Department of Health and Human Services, Public Health Service, Office of Minority Health Resource Center (OMH-RC), was established by the U.S. Department of Health and Human Services, Office of Minority Health (OMH) in October 1987. The Resource Center maintains information on health-related resources, targeting Asian/Pacific Islanders, blacks, Hispanics/Latinos, and Native Americans, available at the federal, state, and local levels. The activities of the OMH-RC concentrate on the following topics: cancer, chemical dependency, diabetes, heart disease and stroke, homicide/suicide, infant mortality, and unintentional injury. The OMH-RC is available to answer requests from consumers and professionals. Bilingual staff are available to assist Spanish-speaking requestors. It offers sources of free and low-cost services and material. The OMH-RC maintains a computerized database of minority health-related materials, organizations, and programs which concentrate on the minority health priority areas and associated risk factors. It has established a network of professionals active in a variety of disciplines that can provide expert technical assistance to minority-based community organizations, voluntary groups, and individuals. Certain services are available in Spanish. Referral services are offered.

Publications

The OMH-RC has prepared a series of fact sheets entitled "Closing the Gap."

MOLD

See under Allergy.

MOUTH

See Dry Mouth (Xerostomia) on page 296.

MULTIPLE SCLEROSIS (MS)

Multiple sclerosis involves a degeneration of myelin, the protective coverings of nerves in the brain and spinal cord. Because myelin is so widespread in the body, the symptoms of multiple sclerosis may manifest in many ways. It begins with a vague, brief symptom that clears up within a few days or weeks. Such symptoms may include a tingling, numbness, or weakness in a limb or a sudden loss of vision. This type of symptom may be produced after a hot bath or in hot weather. For some people there are repeated attacks, and recovery becomes less complete with some residual disability. For a small group, the disease never recurs after the initial episode.

MULTIPLE SCLEROSIS ASSOCIATION OF AMERICA *1-609-858-3211*
601-05 White Horse Pike *1-800-822-4MSA 24-hour hotline*
Oaklyn, NJ 08107

Purpose This national health care organization is dedicated to providing services and programs to assist those with multiple sclerosis. It provides peer counseling, support groups, free loan of therapeutic equipment, a bimonthly newsletter, social and group activities, barrier-free housing, and referrals to physicians and self-help groups.

Publications

Motivator, MS newsletter.

MS and Sexuality, Sensuality.

MS Maintenance.

MSAA Services Brochure.

SSI.

Support Groups.

Understanding MS.

MULTIPLE SCLEROSIS FOUNDATION (MSF) *1-305-776-6805*
6350 N. Andrews Avenue *1-305-938-8708*
Fort Lauderdale, FL 33309 *1-800-441-7055*

Purpose The Foundation offers support services and information distribution on holistic and medical care options for those whose lives have been affected by multiple sclerosis. It also provides grants for research at Universities and clinics throughout the country. MSF does not endorse any one health care approach but informs people on the options for treatments and offers support. It will refer to physicians and self-help groups. Information is obtained through library searches and contacts with organizations and health care professionals.

Publications

MS Focus, quarterly newsletter focusing on grants awarded and holistic care options, interviews, and research updates.

New Hope, Real Help, by John Pageler, an MS patient's story about how he coped with a diagnosis of MS and his suggestions for diet and nutrition.

NATIONAL INSTITUTE OF NEUROLOGICAL DISORDERS AND STROKE (NINDS) *1-301-496-5751*
Building 31, Room 8A06
Bethesda, MD 20892

Publication

Multiple Sclerosis, NIH Pub. No. 81-75.

NATIONAL INSTITUTES OF HEALTH (NIH) *1-301-496-2563*
Office of Clinical Center Communications
Building 10, Room 1C255
Bethesda, MD 20892

Publication

Multiple Sclerosis, NIH Pub. No. 90-3015.

MYASTHENIA GRAVIS (MG)

An acquired autoimmune (self-destructive) disease, the initial symptoms of myasthenia gravis are upper eyelid drop, blurred vision, and general weakness and fatigue. There also may be difficulty in swallowing, facial weakness, and slurred nasal speech.

MYASTHENIA GRAVIS FOUNDATION
53 West Jackson Blvd., Suite 660
Chicago, IL 60604

1-312-427-6252
1-800-541-5454

Purpose The Foundation provides literature, support groups, and patient services; sponsors medical symposia; funds research; assists patients as needed; and provides professional literature for physicians and nurses. It refers to physicians in your locale and self-help groups.

Publications
A Manual for the Nurse.
Myasthenia Gravis Foundation Programs.
Physician's Manual.
Practical Guide to Myasthenia Gravis on Diagnosis and Treatment.
Survival Guide Re: Coping with Myasthenia Gravis.

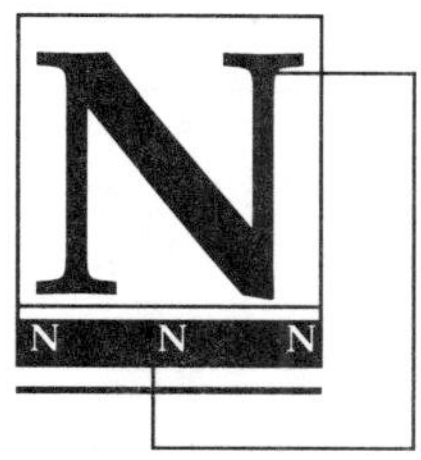

NARCOLEPSY

Narcolepsy involves irresistible attacks of sleep, often with muscular weakness. Attacks occur during waking hours, not only under conditions conducive to drowsiness—after a heavy meal, during a dull lecture—but in inappropriate and even hazardous circumstances.

AMERICAN NARCOLEPSY ASSOCIATION *1-415-788-4793*
P.O. Box 26230
San Francisco, CA 94126-6230

Purpose The Association seeks to improve the lives of people with narcolepsy. It provides information on medication, Social Security, insurance, and support groups for people with narcolepsy. It will also refer to sleep disorder centers.

Publications
American Narcolepsy Association brochure, nontechnical information, Social Security information, American with Disabilities Act information, a quarterly newsletter, and medications information.

NATIONAL INSTITUTE OF NEUROLOGICAL DISORDERS AND STROKE (NINDS) *1-301-496-5751*
Building 31, Room 8A06
Bethesda, MD 20892

Publication
Narcolepsy, NIH Pub. No. 89-1637.

NATIONAL INSTITUTES OF HEALTH (NIH)

Division of Public Information *1-301-496-5787*
Office of Communications
Bethesda, MD 20892

Purpose The NIH is the principal medical research arm of the federal government. It is one of six health agencies of the Public Health Service, a component of the U.S. Department of Health and Human Services. The mission of NIH is to improve the health of the nation by increasing our understanding of the processes underlying human health and by acquiring new knowledge to help prevent, detect, diagnose, and treat disease.

On its 306-acre campus in Bethesda, Maryland, the NIH maintains hundreds of research laboratories and associated office facilities; a 540-bed research hospital—the Warren G. Magnuson Clinical Center—and its adjoining clinic; the National Library of Medicine, the world's largest repository of biomedical information and a national center for biomedical communications; and the Fogarty International Center, which is the focal point for coordination of NIH international relationships and the support of worldwide programs.

The NIH funds nearly 40 percent of all biomedical research and development in the United States.

NATIONAL CANCER INSTITUTE (NCI) *1-301-496-5583*
Office of Cancer Communications *1-800-4-CANCER*
Bethesda, MD 20892

Purpose The NCI is the primary federal agency in cancer research, leading and coordinating all federal activities in this area and providing support to the cancer-fighting work of state and local governments, industries, voluntary health agencies, and other organizations. In addition, the Institute

- Conducts cancer research in its own laboratories
- Supports cancer research and a cancer control program through research grants and contracts
- Supports training of new cancer researchers
- Collects and disseminates information on cancer to researchers, health professionals, and the public

NCI supports cancer research by investigators at universities, medical centers, and institutions throughout the country. NCI also conducts a vigorous intramural research program in the areas of cancer cause and prevention, cancer detection and diagnosis, and cancer treatment and rehabilitation.

NCI provides a variety of information to basic and clinical researchers, health professionals, and the public. NCI publishes the *Journal of the National Cancer Institute* and a number of brochures on the various forms of cancer. In addition, the Cancer Information Service, located in 20 cities around the United States, relays the latest cancer information to patients, the public, and health professionals through its toll-free number and community outreach programs.

NATIONAL EYE INSTITUTE (NEI) *1-301-496-5248*
Information Office
Building 31, Room 6B32
Bethesda, MD 20892

Purpose The NEI fosters research to gain knowledge and understanding of the normal function of the eye and visual system, the pathology of visual disorder, and the basic science underlying vision. To this end, the Institute

- Supports—through grants, fellowships, and contracts—research and research training aimed at improving the prevention, diagnosis, and treatment of visual disorders
- Conducts laboratory and clinical research in its own facilities and fosters statistical and epidemiological studies of visual disorders in human populations
- Promotes research to rehabilitate the visually handicapped
- Encourages application of research discoveries to clinical practice
- Heightens public awareness of vision problems
- Cooperates with voluntary organizations in related activities

Approximately 85 percent of NEI's appropriated funds are used to support investigators at U.S. universities and medical schools. Primary areas of support include retinal and choroidal disease, corneal diseases, cataract, glaucoma, and sensory and motor disorders of vision.

NATIONAL HEART, LUNG, AND BLOOD INSTITUTE EDUCATION PROGRAMS (NHLBI) *1-301-951-3260*
Information Center
Information Specialist
4733 Bethesda Avenue, Suite 530
Bethesda, MD 20814

For information on disorders of the heart, lung, and blood, contact:

Communications and Public Information Branch
Office of Prevention, Education, and Control
NHLBI, NIH
Bethesda, MD 20892
1-301-496-4239

Purpose The NHLBI plans, conducts, and supports a coordinated program of basic and clinical research, clinical trials, and demonstration and education programs relating to the causes, methods of diagnosis, treatment, and prevention of heart, blood vessel, and lung and blood diseases.

- The Division of Heart and Vascular Disease plans and directs the NHLBI's grant, contract, and training programs concerned with atherosclerosis, hypertension, cerebral vascular disease, coronary heart disease, peripheral vascular disease, arrhythmia, heart failure and shock, congenital and rheumatic heart disease, cardiomyopathies and infections of the heart, and circulatory assistance.
- The Division of Lung Diseases guides and supports research into lung disorders, encompassing basic and targeted research in lung structure and function, chronic obstructive lung disease, pediatric pulmonary disease, fibrotic and immunologic interstitial lung disease, respiratory failure, and pulmonary vascular disease.

- The Division of Blood Diseases and Resources, through grants, contracts, and training programs, supports and directs research in the bleeding and clotting disorders, sickle cell disease and other disorders of the red blood cell, and the efficient and safe use of blood and blood products. The Division manages the National Marrow Donor Program.
- The Division of Epidemiology and Clinical Applications plans and directs epidemiological studies, clinical trials, basic and applied research, and projects for disease prevention and health promotion in heart, vascular, pulmonary, and blood diseases.
- The 18 Bethesda-based laboratories of the Division of Intramural Research conduct a variety of basic and clinical studies on the cardiopulmonary, blood, and endocrine systems in health and disease.

The Office of Prevention, Education, and Control is the Institute's technology transfer arm, relaying the results of heart, lung, and blood research to health care professionals, their patients, and the public. The Institute administers five major education programs: National High Blood Pressure Education, National Cholesterol Education, National Blood Resource Education, National Asthma Education, and Smoking Education.

NATIONAL INSTITUTE OF ALLERGY AND INFECTIOUS DISEASES (NIAID) *1-301-496-5717*
Office of Communications
9000 Rockville Pike
Bldg. 31, Room 7A32
Bethesda, MD 20892

Purpose The NIAID conducts and supports research on allergic, immunologic, and infectious diseases. Among NIAID's major areas of emphasis are the following:

- *Immunologic diseases.* Scientists doing basic research are examining how the immune system functions, and clinical investigators are using this knowledge to find ways to treat immunologic diseases, including allergies and asthma, autoimmune disorders, and immune deficiency diseases.
- *Genetics and transplantation.* By determining the genetic mechanisms of the immune response, scientists will be able to develop techniques for tissue typing and more effective ways to prevent infectious diseases.
- *Vaccine development.* Advances in molecular biology and immunology have enabled scientists to design new approaches to developing vaccines to prevent infectious diseases.
- *Antiviral research.* NIAID supports an extensive program aimed at developing and testing antiviral drugs for diseases such as hepatitis B, herpes infections, and cytomegalovirus infection.
- *Sexually transmitted diseases.* NIAID-supported scientists are working to develop better diagnostic tests, improved treatments, and effective vaccines for these widespread and often devastating diseases.
- *Acquired immunodeficiency syndrome.* Studies are underway to develop effective ways to treat and prevent human immunodeficiency virus (HIV) infection and

AIDS, to define the natural history of the disease, and to identify risk factors for HIV infection.

- *Parasitic and fungal diseases.* Scientists at NIAID and at research institutions around the world are developing vaccines and improved therapies for such tropical diseases as malaria, filariasis, and trypanosomiasis.

NATIONAL INSTITUTE OF ARTHRITIS AND MUSCULOSKELETAL AND SKIN DISEASES (NIAMSD) *1-301-496-8188*
Office of Scientific and Health Communications
Building 31, Room 4C05
Bethesda, MD 20892

Purpose The National Institute of Arthritis and Musculoskeletal and Skin Diseases leads, coordinates, stimulates, conducts, and supports the national biomedical research effort on a broad range of diseases and long-lasting, disabling conditions in the fields of rheumatology, orthopedics, bone and mineral metabolism, muscle biology, and dermatology.

Through its extramural program, NIAMSD supports a wide spectrum of basic and clinical research and research training at universities and medical centers throughout the country. Grantees investigate the normal structure and function of the joints, muscles, bones, and skin, as well as disease, such as (1) arthritis and related rheumatic disorders, including rheumatoid arthritis, osteoarthritis, lupus, scleroderma, Lyme disease, ankylosing spondylitis, and juvenile arthritis; (2) musculoskeletal and bone disorders, such as osteoporosis, Paget's disease, heritable connective tissue disorders, and sports injuries; and (3) skin diseases, such as psoriasis, epidermolysis bullosa, ichthyosis, vitiligo, acne, and alopecia areata.

The Institute's intramural research program focuses on

- Muscle biochemistry, biophysics, and ultrastructure
- Molecular genetics and membrane and receptor biochemistry
- Molecular genetics, virology, and cellular immunology of autoimmune diseases
- Ultrastructure of viruses
- Developmental biology and repair of bone matrix
- Expression and structure of proteins of the epidermis.

Clinical research is concentrated in the areas of systemic lupus erythematosus, rheumatoid arthritis, and polymyositis.

NIAMSD also carries out information, education, and prevention activities through the Office of Prevention, Epidemiology, and Clinical Applications, the Office of Scientific and Health Communications; and the National Arthritis and Musculoskeletal and Skin Diseases Information Clearinghouse. These programs serve the important function of communicating research results to the public and disseminating to health professionals those biomedical research efforts to improve the diagnosis, treatment, and prevention of osteoporosis. The Institute sponsors basic research on bone biology and bone metabolism: specialized centers of research on osteoporosis and educational programs.

NATIONAL INSTITUTE OF CHILD HEALTH AND HUMAN DEVELOPMENT (NICHHD) *1-301-496-5133*
Office of Research Reporting
Building 31
Bethesda, MD 20892

Purpose The NICHHD conducts and supports research on the reproductive, developmental, and behavioral processes that determine the health of children, adults, families, and populations. To accomplish this mission, the Institute administers a multidisciplinary program of research, research training, and public information.

NICHHD has four major components that engage in biomedical and behavioral projects and fundamental and clinical studies. They are

- The Center for Research for Mothers and Children
- The Center for Population Research
- Intramural Research Program
- The Prevention Research Program

The Institute supports research in the reproductive sciences to develop knowledge enabling men and women to regulate their fertility with methods that are safe, effective, and acceptable to various population groups and to overcome problems of infertility.

In population, social, and behavioral sciences, the purpose of Institute-sponsored research is to understand the causes and consequences of population change.

Research for mothers, children, and families is designed to advance knowledge of fetal development, pregnancy, and birth; to identify the prerequisites of optimal growth through infancy, childhood, and adolescence; and to contribute to the prevention and treatment of mental retardation. A major program supports research designed to combat infant mortality. Maternal, adolescent, and pediatric AIDS is receiving increasing attention.

NATIONAL INSTITUTE OF DENTAL RESEARCH (NIDR) *1-301-496-4261*
See also Teeth.
9000 Rockville Pike
Bldg. 31, Room 2C35
Bethesda, MD 20892

Purpose The NIDR is the primary sponsor of dental research and related training in the United States. Its mission is to support studies to establish the causes, develop better treatments, and ultimately find ways to prevent or substantially lower the risk of developing oral disease. The NIDR covers 14 areas of oral health research:

1. Dental caries
2. Periodontal disease
3. Congenital craniofacial malformations

4. Acquired craniofacial defects
5. Dentofacial malrelations
6. Soft tissue disease
7. Craniofacial pain and sensory-motor dysfunction
8. Salivary glands and secretions
9. Mineralized tissues and fluoride studies
10. Pulp biology
11. Nutrition research
12. Behavioral studies
13. Implants, replants, and transplants
14. Restorative materials

Publications

The Extramural Program of the National Institute of Dental Research.
The Intramural Research Program of the National Institute of Dental Research.
The National Institute of Dental Research.

NATIONAL INSTITUTE OF DIABETES AND DIGESTIVE AND KIDNEY DISEASES (NIDDK) *1-301-496-3583*
9000 Rockville Pike
Bldg. 31, Room 9804
Bethesda, MD 20892

Purpose The NIDDK conducts and supports research on many of the most serious diseases affecting the public health. The Institute undertakes both basic and clinical research on diabetes, and endocrine and metabolic disorders, including cystic fibrosis; digestive diseases and nutritional disorders; and kidney and urinary tract diseases and blood disorders.

The Endocrinology Research Program of NIDDK has a strong commitment to the support of research on the bone-active hormones and cytokines. Understanding the mechanism of action and the regulation of bone metabolism by parathyroid hormone, calcitonin, the calciferols, steroids, and growth factors will lead to an awareness of the causes and eventually the cure of many bone diseases, such as osteoporosis.

NATIONAL INSTITUTE OF ENVIRONMENTAL HEALTH SCIENCES (NIEHS) *1-919-541-3345*
Office for Public Information
P.O. Box 12233
Research Triangle Park, NC 27709

Purpose The only component of NIH not located in Bethesda, the NIEHS is headquartered in Research Triangle Park, North Carolina. NIEHS investigates the effects of chemical, physical, and biological environmental agents on human health. The Institute's goal is to provide the scientific information base, advanced methodology, and trained personnel to understand and prevent adverse effects of environmental factors on human health.

The Institute supports training in environmental toxicology pathology, mutagenesis, and epidemiology. NIEHS also funds basic and applied research on the exposure of human and other biological systems to potentially toxic or harmful environmental agents.

In addition, the Institute administers a grant program authorized by the Superfund Amendments and Reauthorization Act of 1986 for health and safety training of workers involved in various aspects of hazardous waste removal.

In its research, the Institute attempts to learn

- How and where potentially harmful agents, particularly chemicals, are released
- How these agents move and possibly change as they move
- The extent of exposure of various population groups
- What effects these agents cause, by themselves and in combination with other environmental factors
- What happens in biological systems after exposure to a hazardous agent
- What diseases are caused or aggravated by environmental factors

Research findings are intended to aid those agencies and organizations, public and private, responsible for developing and instituting regulations, policies, and procedures to prevent and reduce the incidence of environmentally induced diseases.

In rounding out these activities, NIEHS supports efforts to identify hazardous agents before they are released into the environment. These include developing, testing, and validating biological assay systems to predict the toxic effects that might occur in humans.

NATIONAL INSTITUTE OF MENTAL HEALTH (NIMH) *1-301-443-4513*

Information Resources and Inquiries Branch
5600 Fishers Lane, Room 15C-05
Rockville, MD 20857

Purpose The NIMH is the federal agency that supports research nationwide on mental illness and mental health. The Institute's Information Resources and Inquiries Branch (IRIB) responds to information requests from the lay public, clinicians, and the scientific community with a variety of publications. These include printed materials on such subjects as destigmatization of mental illness, schizophrenia, paranoia, depression, bipolar disorder, anxiety and panic disorders, AIDS, obsessive-compulsive disorder, anorexia nervosa and bulimia, and Alzheimer's disease. It distributes information and publications on the Depression/Awareness, Recognition, and Treatment Program (D/ART), an NIMH-sponsored educational program on depressive disorders and their symptoms and treatments.

NATIONAL INSTITUTE OF NEUROLOGICAL AND COMMUNICATIVE DISORDERS AND STROKE (NINCDS)
P.O. Box 5801
Bethesda, MD 20824

1-301-496-5751
1-800-352-9424
Fax 1-301-402-2186

Purpose The NINCDS is America's focal point for support of research on brain and nervous system disorders. Created by the U.S. Congress in 1950, the NINCDS seeks better understanding, diagnosis, treatment, and prevention of neurological disorders. Some key areas of clinical research are

- Alzheimer's disease and related dementias
- Brain imaging, including positron emission tomography (PET) and magnetic resonance imaging (MRI)
- Effects of drugs on the brain
- Epilepsy
- Head and spinal cord injury
- Huntington's disease and other inherited diseases such as Batten's and Gaucher's disease, hereditary ataxias, neurofibromatosis, and dystonias
- Nerve and muscle disorders, including diabetic neuropathy, muscular dystrophy, and amyotrophic lateral sclerosis
- Neuro-AIDS and other infections of the brain
- Pain
- Parkinson's disease
- Sleep and sleep disorders
- Stroke and cerebrovascular disease

Publications

Amyotrophic Lateral Sclerosis, NIH Pub. No. 84-916.
Aphasia, NIH Pub. No. 91-391.
Brain Tumors, NIH Pub. No. 82-504.
Cerebral Palsy, NIH Pub. No. 81-159.
Chronic Pain, NIH Pub. No. 90-2406.
Developmental Speech & Language Disorders, NIH Pub. No. 88-2757.
Dizziness, NIH Pub. No. 86-76.
Epilepsy, NIH Pub. No. 81-156.
Headache, NIH Pub. No. 84-158.
Head Injury, NIH Pub. No. 84-2478.
Multiple Sclerosis, NIH Pub. No. 79-75.
Parkinson's Disease, NIH Pub. No. 83-139.
Shingles (Herpes Zoster), NIH Pub. No. 82-307.
Spina Bifida, NIH Pub. No. 86-309.
Spinal Cord Injury, NIH Pub. No. 81-160.
Stroke, NIH Pub. No. 83-2222.

FACT SHEETS

Batten's Disease, NIH Pub. No. 87-2790.

Creutzfeldt-Jakob Disease, NIH Pub. No. 86-2760.
Friedreich's Ataxia, NIH Pub. No. 82-87.
Huntington's Disease.
Joseph's Disease, NIH Pub. No. 85-2716.
Lipid Storage Diseases, NIH Pub. No. 84-2628.
Mutliple Sclerosis.
Narcolepsy, NIH Pub. No. 89-1637.
Neurofibromatosis, NIH Pub. No. 83-2126.
Positron Emission Tomography, NIH Pub. No. 84-2620.
Special Reports, annual or biennial research updates.
Symptomatic Carotid Endarterectomy Trial.
Tourette Syndrome, NIH Pub. No. 83-2163.
Tuberous Sclerosis, NIH Pub. No. 85-1846.

IN SPANISH

Autismo, NIH *Pub. No. 81-2282.*

NATIONAL INSTITUTE ON AGING (NIA) *1-301-496-1752*
Public Inquiries
Federal Building, Room 6C12
Bethesda, MD 20892

Purpose The National Institute on Aging is charged with the responsibility for the conduct and support of biomedical, social, and behavioral research and training related to the aging process and the diseases and other special problems and needs of the aged. The NIA supports research on osteoporosis and related topics, such as bone loss, falls, and hip fractures, which are major causes of frailty and dependence experienced among the older population.

The Institute is organized into two intramural and three extramural programs that address the wide range of health issues of concern to older adults. The Office of Alzheimer's Disease Research manages the NIH Coordinating Committee on Alzheimer's Disease Research.

The NIA conducts laboratory and clinical research at its intramural Gerontology Research Center in its Laboratory of Neurosciences. The GRC's Baltimore Longitudinal Study of Aging, a long-term study initiated in 1958 and involving approximately 1,000 male and female volunteers, is helping scientists learn to differentiate between changes that are due primarily to aging and those attributable to disease or environmental influences.

The Intramural Epidemiology, Demography, and Biometry Program conducts and supports research in the epidemiology of health and disease and the demographic, social, and economic factors that affect the health status of older people.

The extramural Biomedical Research and Clinical Medicine Program supports studies that focus on diseases associated with increasing age and the basic mechanisms involved in the aging process. The program funds research and training on molecular and cellular biology, genetics, immunology, exercise physiology, rehabilitation, nutrition, endocrinology, pharmacology, and geriatric medicine.

The Behavioral and Social Research Program's extramural research focuses on how people grow old and on older people's interrelationships with their environments, families, and other social groups. The program emphasizes research on promoting healthy and productive functions in the middle and later years.

The extramural Neuroscience and Neuropsychology of Aging Program supports research on the structure and function of the aging nervous system and the behavioral manifestations of the aging brain. Of special interest is the study of Alzheimer's disease, including its causes, diagnosis, treatment, incidence, and prevalence.

NATIONAL INSTITUTE ON DEAFNESS AND OTHER COMMUNICATION DISORDERS (NIDOCD)
Program Planning and Health Reports Branch
Building 31, Room 1B62
Bethesda, MD 20892

1-301-496-7243
1-301-402-0018 TDD

Purpose In October 1988 NIDOCD became the thirteenth institute mandated by Congress within the National Institutes of Health. The NIDOCD conducts and supports research and training on normal mechanisms as well as disorders of hearing and other communication processes, including diseases affecting hearing, balance, smell, taste, voice, speech, and language.

The NIDOCD performs a wide range of research in its own laboratories and administers a program of research grants, individual and institutional research training awards, career development awards, center grants, and contracts to public and private research institutions and organizations. The Institute also conducts and supports research and training that is related to disease prevention and health promotion.

The NIDOCD addresses special biomedical and behavioral problems that affect people who have communication impairments or disorders. The NIDOCD supports efforts to create devices that substitute for lost and impaired sensory and communication functions.

The legislation that established NIDOCD also directed that the Institute establish the NIDOCD National Information Clearinghouse to collect and disseminate information to health professionals, patients, industry, and the public on research findings related to deafness and other communication disorders.

NEUROFIBROMATOSIS

Two genetically distinct forms of neurofibromatosis have been identified: *Neurofibromatosis-1* (NF-1), formerly called von Recklinghausen's disease or peripheral neurofibromatosis, is estimated to occur in 1 of 4,000 births NF-1 is characterized by

- Multiple cafe-au-lait colored spots on the skin
- Tumors of varying sizes on or under the skin
- Lisch nodules on the iris of the eyes
- Freckling in the underarm or groin area
- Optic glioma
- Nerve tumors

Neurofibromatosis-2 (NF-2), commonly called central form, is estimated to occur in one of 50,000 births. It is characterized by

- Tumors developing in the eighth cranial nerve complex affecting the auditory nerves often resulting in deafness and balance problems
- Tumors in the brain or spinal cord
- Cataracts of the eye occurring at any age
- Signs of the disorder usually appearing in puberty and beyond

NATIONAL INSTITUTE OF NEUROLOGICAL DISORDERS AND STROKE (NINDS) *1-301-496-5751*
Building 31, Room 8A06
Bethesda, MD 20892

Publication

Neurofibromatosis, NIH Pub. No. 83-2126.

NEUROFIBROMATOSIS, INC. *1-301-577-8984 24 hours*
3401 Woodridge Court
Mitchellville, MD 20721-2817

Purpose This is a voluntary organization that provides information on the neurofibromatoses and related conditions, makes referrals to physicians and medical centers familiar with the conditions, and stimulates research. The organization provides meetings with interpreters for the deaf, peer counseling, referrals to research projects, and speakers on NF-1 and NF-2 and reviews from a layperson's point of view publications dealing with rare conditions, genetic disorders, and voluntary organizations, as well as the neurofibromatoses and related conditions.

Publications

Neurofibromatosis, reprint of 1987 NIH Consensus Development Conference State with four year update which gives diagnostic criteria and general management recommendations for NF-1 and NF-2.

NF, Inc., Serving NF Families, a fact sheet on NF-1 and NF-2 and NF, Inc.

How NF Can Affect the Body, a diagram of a body signifying how NF can physically affect the person with NF. Also available in Spanish.

NEUROLOGY

More than 600 neurological disorders affect the brains and nerves of an estimated 50 million Americans. The disorders cost more than $150 billion in medical expenses and lost productivity. They include nerve and muscle disorders such as diabetic neuropathy, muscular dystrophy, and amyotrophic lateral sclerosis. They also include Parkinson's disease, sleep disorders, stroke, multiple sclerosis, Alzheimer's disease, developmental disorders including autism, dyslexia, attention deficit disorder, cerebral palsy, and spina bifida.

NEUROSURGERY

Neurological surgery is the specialty that deals with surgery of the brain and spinal cord; the control of pain, and the management of head trauma and spinal trauma.

AMERICAN ASSOCIATION OF NEUROLOGICAL SURGEONS *1-708-692-9500*
22 S. Washington St.
Park Ridge, IL 60068

Purpose The Association seeks the advancement of and the pursuit of excellence in neurological surgery and related sciences. It answers inquiries but does not refer to specialists or self-help groups.

Publications
What Is a Brain Tumor?
What Is a Slipped Disc?
What Is a Stroke?
What Is Neurosurgery?

NOSEBLEEDS

Nosebleeds can occur spontaneously as a result of injury, from diseases such as high blood pressure, from strenuous activity, colds, or exposure to high altitudes.

AMERICAN ACADEMY OF OTOLARYNGOLOGY *1-703-836-4444*
HEAD AND NECK SURGERY (AAOHNS) *Fax 1-703-683-5100*
One Prince Street
Alexandria, VA 22314

Publication
Send a stamped, self-addressed envelope for
Nosebleeds, Care & Prevention.

NURSING HOMES

When it becomes necessary to place a loved one in a long-term care facility, an educated choice must be made. Good nursing home accommodations are in short supply and expensive.

NATIONAL INSTITUTE ON AGING (NIA) *1-301-496-1752*
Public Inquiries
Federal Building, Room 6C12
Bethesda, MD 20892

Publication
When You Need a Nursing Home.

NUTRITION

See also Diet.

Eating the right thing is essential for the maintenance or restoration of health. But what is the "right thing"? There is much confusing information being fed to us. Not everyone should follow the same diet. Some need more protein than others, and some have to be careful of the amount. At any given time, millions of Americans are on a reducing diet, some even to the point of starvation. There are experts who can answer your questions about nutrition.

AGRICULTURAL RESEARCH SERVICE *1-301-344-2403*
National Visitor Center
Education Program
Building 302
Beltsville, MD 20705

Contacts For Assistance

Local Contacts (listed in your telephone directory)	*Ask for the*
Health Department (city, county or state)	*Public health nutritionist*
Extension Service (country or state)	*Home economist*
Hospital (any one)	*Registered dietitian*
College or University	*Nutrition instructor or dietitian*
Dept. of Home Economics, Nutrition, Dietetics, Food Science	

ALLIANCE FOR FOOD AND FIBER *1-800-266-0200*
Messages can be heard 24 hours but calls are returned Monday through Friday, 9 A.M. to 5 P.M. PST.

Purpose A project of California produce growers' trade associations, the Alliance provides a choice of six recorded food safety messages, including one about the role of government in monitoring the food supply and another on how to safely handle food at home. For answers to specific inquiries, you can bypass the recorded messages and have your questions recorded. After consulting with either a staff nutritionist or a food safety specialist, a staff member will return your call the next business day.

ASTHMA AND ALLERGY FOUNDATION OF AMERICA (AAFA) *1-202-265-0265*
1717 Massachusetts Ave., N.W., Suite 305
Washington, D.C. 20036

DIABETES EDUCATION CENTER
St. Louis Park Medical Center Research Foundation
4959 Excelsior Blvd.
Minneapolis, MN 55416

Publications
Convenience Food Lists.
Adding Fiber to Your Diet.

FOOD AND DRUG ADMINISTRATION (FDA) *1-301-433-3170*
Office of Consumer Affairs (HFE-88)
5600 Fishers Lane
Rockville, MD 20857

GLUTEN INTOLERANCE GROUP *1-206-854-9606*
26604 Dover Court
Kent, WA 98031
Check for what is available.

HCF NUTRITION RESEARCH FOUNDATION, INC. *1-606-276-3119*
Manager, P.O. Box 22124
Lexington, KY 40522

Purpose The HCF Nutrition Research Foundation is a nonprofit, public foundation founded in 1979. HCF promotes nutrition as a choice for better health, as well as advocating a healthful life-style, which includes regular exercise, not smoking, and stress management. An HCF nutrition plan helps in the prevention and treatment of conditions such as diabetes, high cholesterol, heart disease, high blood pressure, obesity, and cancer by increasing fiber in the diet. The Foundation disseminates information through seminars, public forums, and personal contacts.

HUMAN NUTRITION INFORMATION SERVICE/USDA *1-301-436-8498*
Public Affairs Staff
6505 Belcrest Rd.
Hyattsville, MD 20782

KELLOGG COMPANY
P.O. Box 3447
Dept. M-1
Battle Creek, MI 49016-3447

Publications

Fiber for a Healthy Life, recipes and information about fiber and health.

Wheat Bran: News About Dietary Fiber and Cancer Prevention, specific information about diet and cancer prevention plus recipes.

MEAT AND POULTRY HOTLINE *1-800-535-4555*
1-202-477-3333 in Washington, D.C.
Weekdays 10 A.M. to 4 P.M. EST

Purpose The Hotline provides information on proper handling, preparation, storing and cooking of meat, poultry, and eggs. It also answers questions about the safe cooking of poultry and meat in microwave ovens.

NATIONAL CENTER FOR NUTRITION AND DIETETICS (NCND) *1-800-366-1655*
(formerly American Dietetic Association)
216 West Jackson Boulevard, Suite 800
Chicago, IL 60606-6996

Purpose The NCND is the public education initiative of the American Dietetic Association and its foundation. It desseminates sound, objective, and timely nutrition information to the public. You can call 24 hours a day, 7 days a week, and choose messages on various topics (touch-tone phones only). The subjects change monthly. You can also speak with a registered dietician from 10 A.M. to 5 P.M. EST, Monday through Friday. In addition, the NCND provides reference services, including literature searches through the Nutrition InfoCenter. Referrals are made to registered dietitians.

Publications

A wide variety of food and nutrition brochures and fact sheets are available.

Eat Right America, a pamphlet containing information about calculating the fat content of foods and tips on cutting down on fat.

NATIONAL CENTER FOR RESEARCH RESOURCES (NCRR) *1-301-496-5545*
Westwood Building, Room 857
Bethesda, MD 20892

Publication

Recent Advances in Clinical Nutrition: The Role of the NIH-Supported General Clinical Research Centers.

NATIONAL HEALTH INFORMATION CLEARINGHOUSE *1-800-336-4797*
P.O. Box 1133 *1-703-522-2390 (in Virginia)*
Washington, D.C. 20013

For food companies, grocery chains, and restaurant franchises, contact the company's consumer affairs department concerning nutrient, additive, and caloric content of their products. Check food labels for addresses.

NATIONAL HEART, LUNG, AND BLOOD INSTITUTE (NHLBI) *1-301-496-4236*
Building 31, Room 4A21
Bethesda, MD 20892

Publication

Nutrition and Your Health: Dietary Guidelines for Americans, Home and Garden Bulletin No. 232.

NATIONAL INSTITUTE ON AGING (NIA) INFORMATION OFFICE
Building 31, Room 5c35
Bethesda, MD 20205

Publications

Fact sheets available in large print:
Be Sensible About Salt.
Dietary Supplements: More Is Not Always Better.
Hints for Shopping, Cooking and Enjoying Meals.
Nutrition: A Lifelong Concern.

NUTRITIONAL INFORMATION CENTER *1-212-746-1617*
515 East 71st St. Suite 904
New York, NY 10021

ODPHP HEALTH INFORMATION CENTER *1-800-336-4797*
P.O. Box 1133 *1-202-429-9091 (in Washington, D.C.)*
Washington, D.C. 20013

RICE COUNCIL OF AMERICA *1-713-270-6699*
P.O. Box 740121
Houston, TX 77274

Publications

Please send stamped, self-addressed envelope for:

The Food Sensitivity Series: Food Sensitivity, Lactose Intolerance, Gluten Intolerance.

Light, Lean and Low Fat: Recipes (30% or less of calories from fat).

Sports Sense—a Guide to Good Eating and Exercise plus Healthful Recipes.

Tasty Rice Recipes . . . for Those with Allergies.

U.S. DEPARTMENT OF AGRICULTURE *1-301-436-8617*
Nutrition Monitoring Division
Human Nutrition Information Service
Federal Building, Room 304A
Hyattsville, MD 20782

WHEAT FOODS COUNCIL *1-303-694-5828*
5500 S. Quebec, Suite 111
Englewood, CO 80111

Purpose The Council engages in nutrition education, particularly about grain-related nutrition questions.

Publication

Facts About Fiber, a brochure about the kinds of fiber and fiber values for common food.

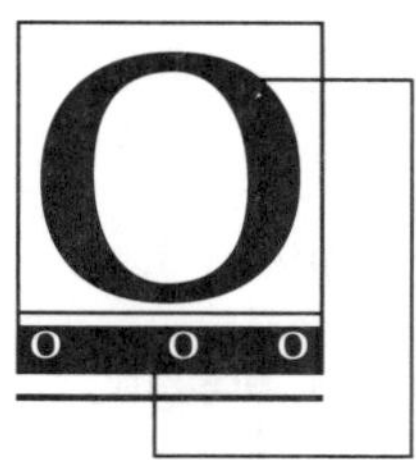

OBESITY

See Diet.

OBSESSIVE COMPULSIVE DISORDER

See under Mental Health.

OBSTETRICS

See Pregnancy.

OCCUPATIONAL HEALTH

The cause and effect between occupation and health are becoming more evident and new methods of investigation and communication are used. In the United States, there are regulations that require safe working conditions for employees.

AMERICAN INDUSTRIAL HYGIENE ASSOCIATION *1-216-873-AIHA*
P.O. Box 8390
345 White Pond Drive
Akron, OH 44320

Purpose The Association is a professional society for those practicing industrial hygiene in industry, government, labor, academic institutions, and independent organizations. Its goal is to keep workers, their families, and the community healthy and safe. It is the industrial hygienist's job to help ensure that federal, state, and local laws and regulations are followed in the work environment.

NATIONAL INSTITUTE FOR OCCUPATIONAL SAFETY AND HEALTH (NIOSH) *1-513-533-8236*
Hazards Evaluations and Technical Assistance Branch (R-9)
U.S. Department of Health and Human Services
4676 Columbia Parkway
Cincinnati, OH 45226

Purpose Congress set up this Institute in 1970 to play a key role in helping to protect workers and their health on the job. The agency was to conduct occupational health research; to inspect manufacturer's plants at employer's and worker's requests, and for its own studies; and to recommend standards for safe exposure to hazardous substances. NIOSH is supposed to work closely with OSHA, the organization responsible for settling the legally permitted exposures to hazards in the workplace. NIOSH, through its investigations into plant conditions and studies of already available data, provides OSHA with the scientific background needed to determine these rules. When a workplace crisis arises, the two agencies often work in tandem to find out how the workers were harmed and to help the industry correct the problem.

OCCUPATIONAL SAFETY AND HEALTH ADMINISTRATION (OSHA) *1-202-523-8148*
U.S. Department of Labor
200 Constitution Ave., N.W.
Washington, D.C. 20210

Purpose OSHA is an agency in the U.S. Department of Labor that establishes workplace safety and health regulations. Many states have their own OSHA programs. This organization has been able to enact human exposure standards for a relatively small number of chemicals in use in the workplace. The Supreme Court ruled that OSHA inspectors cannot conduct surprise health and safety checks at workplaces without a warrant.

OCCUPATIONAL THERAPY

Trained personnel in this field can help make a patient more independent by showing the patient how to use mechanical aids to perform a great many activities of daily living such as bathing and dressing. The therapist may also enable a physically challenged patient to obtain or return to a job.

AMERICAN OCCUPATIONAL THERAPY ASSOCIATION (AOTA) *1-301-948-9626*
1383 Piccard Drive, Suite 300 *1-800-366-9799*
Rockville, MD 20850 *Fax 1-301-948-5512*

Purpose AOTA's CareerLine exists to provide individuals with information about careers in occupational therapy, including information on colleges and universities that offer occupational therapy training, information on scholarships, loans, and other financial aid.

Publications
List of occupational therapist programs.
Posters.

Brochures
Financing Your Occupational Therapy Education.
Occupational Therapy Careers: Caring People Choose.
Occupational Therapy Careers: Caring, Sharing, Connecting.
Occupational Therapy Education Programs.
Occupational Therapy Scholarships, Loans and Financial Aid.
Your Future in Occupational Therapy.

ORGAN TRANSPLANTS

Surgery to replace some damaged body organs with healthy ones is now routine, except to the person, of course, undergoing the transplant. Thousands of such operations are done every year. Health replacements come either from people who have consented or whose surviving relations consent to the medical use of the parts of the body after death, or from living donors who are usually relatives of the recipients.

AMERICAN COUNCIL ON TRANSPLANTATION *1-800-ACT-GIVE*
P.O. Box 1709
Alexandria, VA 22313-1709

LIVING BANK *1-800-528-2971*
P.O. Box 6725
Houston, TX 77265

ORTHODONTISTS

See Dentistry.

ORTHOMOLECULAR THERAPY

See Mental Health.

ORTHOPEDICS

The surgical and medical specialty concerned with correction of deformities, diseases, accidents and disorders of body parts that move us about—limbs, bones, joints, muscles and tendons.

SHRINER'S HOSPITAL
2900 Rocky Point Drive
Tampa, FL 33607

Purpose This organization provides free orthopedic care for children.

OSTEONECROSIS

See under Arthritis Foundation.

OSTEOPATHIC MEDICINE

The word "osteopath" is derived from the Greek words *osteo*, meaning "bone" and *pathos*, meaning "suffering." Osteopathic physicians are from a school of medicine based upon a concept of the normal body as a vital machine capable, when in correct adjustment, of making its own remedies against infections and other toxic conditions; practitioners use the diagnostic and therapeutic measures of conventional medicine in addition to manipulative measures.

AMERICAN OSTEOPATHIC ASSOCIATION (AOA) *1-312-280-5800*
142 E. Ontario St. *1-800-621-1773*
Chicago, IL 60611

Purpose Across the nation, the AOA, which represents more than 32,000 osteopathic physicians, promotes the public health, encourages scientific research, and acts as the accrediting agency for osteopathic medicine and osteopathic medical education. It also provides a physician referral brochure.

Publications

Osteopathic Medicine, a brochure that provides general information on osteopathic medicine, including statistics.

Osteopathic Medical Education, a brochure that explains the education and training of osteopathic physicians.

What Is a D.O.? a brochure that explains the similarities and differences between osteopathic physicians (D.O.s) and allopathic physicians (M.D.s).

OSTEOPOROSIS

See also Arthritis.

A condition characterized by low bone mass and an increased susceptibility to bone fractures. Over a million bone fractures each year, widespread disability and billions of dollars in health care expenses occur because of osteoporosis.

NATIONAL INSTITUTES OF HEALTH (NIH) *1-301-496-2563*
Office of Clinical Center Communications
Building 10, Room 1C255
Bethesda, MD 20892

Publication
Osteoporosis, NIH Pub. No. 89-2983.

OSTOMY

An ostomy is an artificial opening into the urinary or intestinal tract or the windpipe that is made to allow waste or air to pass through.

UNITED OSTOMY ASSOCIATION, INC. (UOA) *1-714-660-8624*
36 Executive Park, Suite 120 *1-800-826-0826*
Irvine, CA 92714

Purpose The United Ostomy Association was formed in 1962 to help ostomy patients return to normal living through mutual aid and moral support, education in proper ostomy care and management, exchange of ideas, assistance in improving ostomy equipment and supplies, advancement of knowledge of gastrointestinal diseases, cooperation with other organizations having common purposes, exhibits at medical and public meetings, and public education about ostomy. Local chapters have medical advisory boards consisting of medical-professional personnel trained in ostomy care and use of equipment. Trained members often visit ostomy patients in hospitals and in their homes to offer moral support and assistance. Monthly meetings provide information on adjusting to living with an ostomy, ileostomy, colostomy, urostomy, and related surgeries. It does not refer to physicians.

Publications
Publications list.

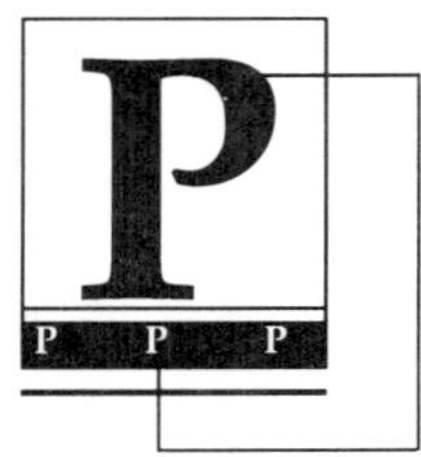

Paget's Disease

Paget's disease is a chronic skeletal disorder that may result in enlarged and deformed bones in one or more regions of the skeleton. It is second only to osteoporosis in the frequency of its occurrence. Although Paget's is often symptomless, some patients experience bone deformity or bone pain, especially in the back and joints. Headaches and hearing loss are common symptoms when the disease affects the skull. The cause of Paget's disease is unknown, but treatments are available to manage it.

National Center for Research Resources (NCRR) *1-301-496-5545*
Westwood Building, Room 857
Bethesda, MD 20892

Publication
Researching the Cause and Treatment of Paget's Disease of Bone.

National Institute of Arthritis and Musculoskeletal and Skin Diseases (NIAMSD) *1-301-496-8188*
Building 31, Room 4C05
Bethesda, MD 20892

Publication
Understanding Paget's Disease, NIH Pub. No. 85-2241.

Paget's Disease Foundation *1-718-596-1043*
165 Cadman Plaza East *Fax 1-718-802-1039*
Brooklyn, NY 11201

Purpose The Foundation's program and services include patient education and assistance, public education, professional education, and research advocacy. One of the services most emphasized is the referral of patients to physicians who treat Paget's disease.

Publications
Questions and Answers About Paget's Disease.
Update, a newsletter published three times a year that reports current information about Paget's disease.

PAIN

Pain is the most frequent cause of suffering and disables more people than cancer or heart disease. According to the Bristol-Meyers Squibb Unrestricted Pain Research Grants Program, almost 90 million Americans are in chronic pain at some time, and many more suffer from acute pain at various times. Headache, backache, and arthritis are the three leading causes of pain in the United States. Chronic pain costs the U.S. economy an estimated $90 billion a year. Lost workdays range from a few days per year for headache sufferers to weeks and even months for those with back, arthritis, cancer, and other pain conditions. The field of pain research is a growing specialty.

AMERICAN CHRONIC PAIN ASSOCIATION (ACPA) *1-916-632-0922*
P.O. Box 850
Rocklin, CA 95677

Purpose A nonprofit organization with over 550 chapters in the United States, Canada, Australia, New Zealand, Mexico, and Russia, the ACPA provides a support system for those suffering with chronic pain. In addition, the ACPA offers training in skills and attitudes that have proven effective in helping people deal with chronic pain. ACPA group members seek to exchange the passive role of patient for that of independent person whose pain is kept in proper perspective. The group does not take the place of traditional medical treatment, but works with the medical community to allow group members to take more responsibility for their own recoveries. Membership is an addition to, not a substitute for, medical and professional services the pain person may already have pursued. Referrals are made to accredited pain management programs and ACPA self-help groups when available.

Publication
Free information packet available upon request.

INTERNATIONAL IMAGERY ASSOCIATION (IIA) *1-914-423-9200*
P.O. Box 1046 *Ask for Red Phone*
Bronx, NY 10471

Purpose The Association engages in the study and applications of mental imagery, education, training, and networking through local, national, and international research, clinical, and personal growth problems. The IIA also keeps a liaison with other organizations interested in collaborating on imagery-related issues and projects. The main thrust is psychosomatics. Referrals are made to local practitioners. The Association also helps organize publications of books and periodicals on imagery.

Publications
Publications list. Charges for publications.
Answers inquiries; provides advisory, consulting, reference, literature-searching, abstracting, and indexing services; evaluates and analyzes data; conducts seminars

and workshops; distributes publications; makes referrals to other sources of information. Services are provided free to some users and at cost to others. All are available to anyone.

NATIONAL INSTITUTE OF DENTAL RESEARCH (NIDR) *1-301-496-0394*
Building 10, Room 3C407
Bethesda, MD 20892

Purpose The Pain Research Clinic at NIDR has ongoing studies in the following areas:

- Painful diabetic neuropathies
- Wisdom tooth extraction
- Causalgic-type pain, including temporomandibular disorders

To find out more about these studies and how to become a patient in these studies (at no cost), write or call NIDR.

Publications
Has a number of ongoing studies concerning pain.

NATIONAL INSTITUTE OF NEUROLOGICAL DISORDERS AND STROKE (NINDS) *1-301-496-5751*
Building 31, Room 8A06
Bethesda, MD 20892

Publication
Pain (Chronic), NIH Pub. No. 89-2406.

NATIONAL INSTITUTES OF HEALTH (NIH) *1-301-496-2563*
Office of Clinical Center Communications
Building 10, Room 1C255
Bethesda, MD 20892

Publications
Relieving Pain.
Relief of Chronic Pain, a videotape that can be borrowed.

SCRIPPS CLINIC AND RESEARCH FOUNDATION *1-619-457-6952*
Pain Treatment Center *1-800-382-4357*
9888 Genesee Ave.
La Jolla, CA 92037

Purpose The Center is involved in the diagnosis and treatment of pain patients and research on pain problems as well as the psychological and physiological aspects of pain. Referrals are made to physicians and self-help groups. Free confidential assessment is available.

Publication

Pain Center-Working Together to Change Your Life.

PARKINSON'S DISEASE

See also Tremor.

Parkinson's disease is a chronic, progressive, degenerative disorder of the central nervous system, named after the British physician who first described it in an essay published in 1817. There are estimated to be nearly half a million persons with the condition, the vast majority of them over age 45. Since the disease develops slowly in a most subtle manner, it is often difficult to make a correct diagnosis early in the course of the disorder. The disease may occur and remain dormant until a period of particular stress or simply physical deterioration through aging causes the appearance of symptoms. Symptoms may include tremor, rigidity, difficulty in voluntary movement, and loss of normal postural reflexes. The tremor, of hand, foot, and occasionally head and/or jaw, is less evident during purposeful activity than during rest and characteristically absent during sleep.

AMERICAN PARKINSON DISEASE ASSOCIATION (APDA) *1-718-981-8001*
60 Bay St., Suite 401 *1-800-223-APDA*
Staten Island, NY 10301 *Fax 1-718-981-4399*

Purpose The APDA was founded in 1961 to "ease the burden and find the cure" of Parkinson's disease. It is the largest organization in the United States dedicated to fighting Parkinson's disease and has supported research leading to major breakthroughs in the knowledge and treatment of Parkinson's disease, education, and increasing public awareness. There are 44 information referral centers located in various universities and hospitals across the United States. There are over 80 chapters and over 350 support groups throughout the country.

Publications

Basic Information About Parkinson's Disease, a 4-page brochure.
Be Active, suggested exercises, 25 pages. Also available in Japanese.
Coping with Parkinson's Disease, 88 pages.
Equipment & Suggestions, 19 pages.
How to Start a Parkinson's Disease Community Support Group, 42 pages.
Parkinson's Challenge, 48 pages.
Parkinson's Disease Handbook, 40 pages. Also available in Spanish and Italian.
Speech & Swallowing Problems, 17 pages. Also available in Japanese.

NATIONAL INSTITUTE OF NEUROLOGICAL DISORDERS AND STROKE (NINDS)
Building 31, Room 8A06
Bethesda, MD 20892

1-301-496-5751

Publication

Parkinson's Disease, NIH Pub. No. 83-239.

NATIONAL INSTITUTES OF HEALTH (NIH)
Office of Clinical Center Communications
Building 10, Room 1C255
Bethesda, MD 20892

1-301-496-2563

Publication

Parkinson's Disease: Natural and Drug-Induced Causes, a videotape that can be borrowed.

NATIONAL PARKINSON FOUNDATION
1501 N.W. 9th Ave.
Bob Hope Road
Miami, FL 33136-1494

1-800-327-4545
Includes all United States, Canada, Caribbean-English, and Spanish-speaking operators.
1-800-433-7022 (Florida only)

Purpose The Foundation undertakes research to find the cause and cure of Parkinson's disease. It provides clinical services; physical, occupational, speech, and neuropsychological therapy; drug tests; information; and education and makes referrals to physicians and self-help groups. The Foundation, which celebrated its 35th anniversary, provides most of its services without charge and never refuses any service to a needy Parkinsonian.

Publications

An Example to Us All—One Woman's Story.
Nutritional Considerations.
Parkinson Diets.
Parkinson Handbook.
Parkinson Quarterly Report.
What Every Patient Should Know.
Some of the publications are available in Spanish.

PARKINSON'S EDUCATIONAL PROGRAM USA (PEP)
3900 Birch Street, Room 105
Newport Beach, CA 92660

1-714-250-2975
1-800-344-7872

Purpose PEP USA is a private, nonprofit association that promotes the establishment of Parkinson's support groups, assists the support groups in services they offer, and helps to protect the rights of people with Parkinson's. PEP also educates the public to an understanding of Parkinson's and supports research into the causes and cure for Parkinson's. PEP makes referrals to physicians and self-help groups in a requestor's locale.

Publications

PEP USA Catalog, a 55-page booklet describing books, videotapes, and products the organization has for sale to Parkinson's patients and their families.

PS? a brochure about Parkinson's syndrome.

UNITED PARKINSON FOUNDATION (UPF) *1-312-664-2344*
360 West Superior Street
Chicago, IL 60610

Purpose The United Parkinson Foundation is an international nonprofit organization chartered in the state of Illinois in 1963. The UPF is an unaffiliated, independent entity which derives its support entirely from its membership and the general public. A major portion of operating expenses is allocated to patient services, which include background literature, exercise materials, and regular newsletters sent to all members regardless of the ability of patients/spouses to contribute funds. The office in Chicago is maintained so that members may call or write for a personal response to specific questions. A Medical Advisory Board is accessible for consultation to the staff on such matters and to supervise publication content and preparation. The office maintains an extensive referral service to guide patients to proper clinical care.

Publications

Newsletters are written primarily for patient and family education, for reporting in layperson's language recent advances in research, for answering questions of general interest to members, and for publishing members' suggestions. Additionally, space is offered to unaffiliated local support groups which provide emotional support and social opportunities for patients and their spouses.

PATHOLOGY

See under Laboratory Topics.

PEDIATRICS

See under Children.

PERIODONTAL DISEASE

Adults lose more teeth from gum disease than from dental decay. The problem is common among young adults, and it increases with age. The disease often can be halted before it reaches an advanced stage.

NATIONAL INSTITUTES OF HEALTH (NIH) *1-301-496-2563*
Office of Clinical Center Communications
Building 10, Room 1C255
Bethesda, MD 20892

Publication

Periodontal Disease, a videotape that can be borrowed.

PESTICIDES

These are compounds that are used to kill pests. People who run the greatest danger of poisoning are those whose exposure is highest, such as workers who mix, load, or apply pesticides. However, the general public also faces the possibility of exposure, and children, because of their small size, are more vulnerable than adults to pesticide poisoning.

NATIONAL PESTICIDE TELECOMMUNICATIONS NETWORK *1-806-743-3091*
S-129 Thompson Hall *1-800-858-7378 Hotline*
Texas Tech University Health Sciences Center
Lubbock, TX 79430

Purpose The Network functions as a 24-hour service providing unbiased, factual information on pesticides (insecticides, herbicides, fungicides, mildewcides, etc.). It is a nonprofit organization funded by a grant from the Environmental Protection Agency. The staffers provide information on the chemical, toxicological, and environmental characteristics by phone and by mail. They offer information on health hazards, cleanup, and disposal of pesticides and will, if necessary, refer callers to human and animal poison control centers in their states.

Publications

A Citizen's Guide to Pesticides, general information on safe use, disposal, and storage of pesticides.

NTPN Brochure, describes service.

Recognition and Management of Pesticide Poisonings, a technical manual detailing typical symptoms and treatment of pesticide exposures.

PHOBIAS

See also Anxiety.

A phobia is an abnormal, excessive dread or fear. There are dozens of common phobias, each with its own medical name such as acrophobia, fear of heights and agoraphobia, fear of open places.

NATIONAL INSTITUTES OF HEALTH (NIH) *1-301-496-2563*
Office of Clinical Center Communications
Building 10, Room 1C255
Bethesda, MD 20892

Publication

Phobias and Panic Disorder, a videotape that can be borrowed.

PHOBIA SOCIETY OF AMERICA (PSA)
See Anxiety.

PHYSICAL FITNESS

Your level of physical fitness reflects your general health and your ability to carry out your daily activities. The quantity and quality of exercise to maintain and strengthen your body are important. There are many sports and activities from which to choose. You want to keep moving, but you don't want to hurt yourself, so you should be informed beforehand of the benefits and hazards of the exercises involved before you begin a program.

AEROBICS AND FITNESS FOUNDATION OF AMERICA (AFFA) *1-800-BE FIT 86*
15250 Ventura Blvd., Suite 310
Sherman Oaks, CA 91403

Purpose AFFA is a nonprofit organization committed to promoting, teaching, and researching safe and effective ways to achieve fitness through aerobic exercise. AFFA also promotes fitness to the nation's youth as a positive alternative to substance abuse through SUPERCLASS events, which are hosted by health clubs. The SUPERCLASS events teach aerobics to teens in drug rehabilitation programs.

Publications

Footnotes are information cards published by AFFA to provide educational facts on health and exercise. They are available upon request by calling AFFA.

AMERICAN ALLIANCE FOR HEALTH, PHYSICAL EDUCATION, RECREATION, AND DANCE (AAHPERD) *1-703-476-3400* *Fax 1-703-476-9527*
1900 Association Drive
Reston, VA 22091

Purpose An alliance of voluntary professional associations, members of AAHPERD share a common mission of education and promoting the related areas of health education, safety, physical education, dance, sport, recreation, and leisure services. Answers to questions by phone will be given.

Publications
Brochures on physical education, recreation, and dance.

PRESIDENT'S COUNCIL ON PHYSICAL FITNESS AND SPORTS *1-202-272-3421*
450 Fifth St., N.W., Suite 7103
Washington, D.C. 20001

Purpose The Council serves as a catalyst in the promotion of exercise and physical fitness for all ages and populations and provides information, programs, and research regarding physical fitness.

Publications
Exercise and Weight Control.
Fitness First, fitness tips.
Fitness Fundamentals.
Fitness in the Workplace.
Get Fit, for youngsters.
One Step at a Time, a running, jogging handbook.
Pep Up Your life, for seniors.
Walking for Exercise and Pleasure.

YMCA OF THE USA *1-312-269-1198*
101 N. Wacker Drive
Chicago, IL 60606

Purpose The YMCA seeks to put Christian principles into practice through programs that build healthy body, mind, and spirit for all. It develops materials and training which are used at 2,200 YMCA locations nationwide. Program categories are Aquatics, Active Older Adults, Camping, Child Care, Community Development, Health and Fitness, Sports, Teens, and Volunteers. Health and fitness programs range from basic exercise, physical fitness evaluations, and back exercise programs, to collaboration with the local medical community. Referrals are made to physicians and self-help groups.

Publications
Available through local YMCAs.

PHYSICIANS

You should choose a family doctor before you are sick. A physician who knows you and your medical history is better able to provide rapid diagnosis and therapy when the need arises.

AMERICAN COLLEGE OF PHYSICIANS *1-215-351-2400*
Independence Mall West *1-800-433-9137*
6th Street at Race
Philadelphia, PA 19106-1572

Purpose The nation's largest medical-specialty society, the College works to uphold health care standards through activities in continuing education, health policy analysis, quality assurance, and medical-technology assessment. Its membership includes more than 70,000 primary care physicians and specialists in the various branches of internal medicine. Disciplines within or related to internal medicine include cardiology, gastroenterology, nephrology, endocrinology, hematology, dermatology, allergy and immunology, psychiatry, critical care medicine, geriatrics, and occupational medicine.

Publication

ACP Health Library, a bimonthly patient education series with materials for patients and physicians. The articles help clarify health issues for patients. Recent topics include cholesterol, screening for colorectal cancer, the skin and ultraviolet light, osteoporosis, adult immunization, and smoking cessation.

PNEUMONIA

See National Jewish Center for Immunology and Respiratory Diseases *under* Allergy.

PODIATRISTS

See Feet.

POISON CONTROL

Curiosity may kill cats, as the saying goes, but it also kills many children every year. There are thousands of chemicals in such common household products as cleaning preparations, cosmetics, medicines, pesticides, and hobby materials. If left within the reach of children, these products are potentially lethal. Even adults mistakenly ingest them.

POISON CONTROL CENTERS

The following is a list of the American Association Of Poison Control Centers, certified regional poison centers as of March 1991.

ALABAMA

ALABAMA POISON CONTROL SYSTEMS, INC.
809 University Boulevard East
Tuscaloosa, AL 35401

Emergency Numbers:
1-800-462-0800 (in Alabama only)
1-205-345-0600

CHILDREN'S HOSPITAL OF ALABAMA—
REGIONAL POISON CONTROL CENTER
1600 Seventh Avenue, South
Birmingham, AL 35233-1711

Emergency Numbers:
1-205-933-4050
1-800-292-6678 (in Alabama only)
Fax 1-205-939-9245

ARIZONA

ARIZONA POISON & DRUG INFORMATION CENTER
Arizona Health Sciences Center, Room 3204-K
University of Arizona
1501 N. Campbell Avenue
Tucson, Arizona 85724

Emergency Numbers:
1-602-626-6016
1-800-362-0101 (in Arizona only)

SAMARITAN REGIONAL POISON CENTER
Good Samaritan Medical Center
1130 East McDowell Road, Suite A-5
Phoenix, AZ 85006

Emergency Number
1-602-253-3334

CALIFORNIA

FRESNO REGIONAL POISON CONTROL CENTER
OF FRESNO COMMUNITY
Hospital and Medical Center
P. 0. Box 1232
2832 Fresno and R Streets
Fresno, CA 93715

Emergency Numbers:
1-209-445-1222
1-800-346-5922
(in seven counties only: Fresno, Kern, Kings, Madera, Mariposa, Merced, Tulare)

LOS ANGELES COUNTY MEDICAL ASSOCIATION
REGIONAL POISON CONTROL CENTER
1925 Wilshire Boulevard
Los Angeles, CA 90057

Emergency Numbers:
1-213-484-5151
1-800-77-POISN
(in three counties only: Los Angeles, Santa Barbara and Ventura)

SAN DIEGO REGIONAL POISON CENTER
UCSD Medical Center
225 Dickinson Street
San Diego, CA 92103

Emergency Numbers:
1-619-543-6000
1-800-876-4766
(in two counties only: San Diego and Imperial)

SAN FRANCISCO BAY AREA
REGIONAL POISON CONTROL CENTER
San Francisco General Hospital, Room 1E86
1001 Potrero Avenue
San Francisco, CA 94110

Emergency Numbers:
1-415-476-6600
1-800-523-2222
(for area codes 415 and 707 only)

UCDMC REGIONAL POISON CONTROL CENTER
2315 Stockton Boulevard
Sacramento, CA 95817

Emergency Numbers:
1-916-734-3692
1-800-342-9293 (for some counties only)

COLORADO

ROCKY MOUNTAIN POISON AND DRUG CENTER
645 Bannock Street
Denver, CO 80204-4507

Emergency Numbers:
1-303-629-1123
1-800-332-3073 (in Colorado only)

DISTRICT OF COLUMBIA

NATIONAL CAPITAL POISON CENTER
Georgetown University Hospital
3800 Reservoir Rd., N.W.
Washington, D.C. 20007

Emergency Numbers:
1-202-625-3333
1-202-784-4660 TTY

FLORIDA

FLORIDA POISON INFORMATION CENTER AT THE
TAMPA GENERAL HOSPITAL
P.O. Box 1289
Tampa, FL 33601

Emergency Numbers:
1-813-253-4444
1-800-282-3171 (in Florida only)

GEORGIA

GEORGIA REGIONAL POISON CONTROL CENTER
Grady Memorial Hospital
Box 26066
80 Butler Street, S.E.
Atlanta, GA 30335-3801

Emergency Numbers:
1-404-589-4400
1-800-282-5846 (in Georgia only)
1-404-525-3323 TTY

KENTUCKY

KENTUCKY REGIONAL POISON CENTER OF
KOSAIR CHILDREN'S HOSPITAL
P.O. Box 35070
Louisville, KY 40232-5070

Emergency Numbers:
1-502-589-8222
(in metropolitan Louisville and Southern Indiana only)
1-800-722-5725 (in Kentucky only)

INDIANA

INDIANA POISON CENTER
Methodist Hospital of Indiana
1701 N. Senate Blvd.
Indianapolis, IN 46206

Emergency Numbers:
1-317-929-2323
1-800-382-9097 (in Indiana only)
1-317-929-2336 TTY

MARYLAND

MARYLAND POISON CENTER
20 North Pine Street
Baltimore, MD 21201

Emergency Numbers:
1-301-528-7701
1-800-492-2414 (in Maryland only)

MASSACHUSETTS

MASSACHUSETTS POISON CONTROL SYSTEM
300 Longwood Avenue
Boston, MA 02115

Emergency Numbers:
1-617-232-2120
1-800-682-9211 (in Massachusetts only)

MICHIGAN

BLODGETT REGIONAL POISON CENTER
Blodgett Memorial Medical Center
1840 Wealthy S.E.
Grand Rapids, MI 49506

Emergency Numbers:
1-800-632-2727 (in Michigan only)
1-800-356-3232
1-616-774-7854 TTY

POISON CONTROL CENTER
Children's Hospital
3901 Beaubien Blvd.
Detroit, MI 48201

Emergency Numbers:
1-313-745-5711
1-800-462-6642 (in Michigan only)

MINNESOTA

HENNEPIN REGIONAL POISON CENTER
Hennepin County Medical Center
701 Park Avenue
Minneapolis, MN 55415

Emergency Numbers:
1-612-347-3141
1-612- 337-7474 TTY

MINNESOTA REGIONAL POISON CENTER
St. Paul-Ramsey Medical Center
640 Jackson Street
St. Paul, MN 55101

Emergency Numbers:
1-612-221-2113
1-800-222-1222 (in Minnesota only)

MISSOURI

MISSOURI REGIONAL POISON CENTER
Cardinal Glennon Children's Hospital
1465 South Grand Blvd.
St. Louis, MO 63104

Emergency Numbers:
1-314-772-5200
1-800-392-9111 (in Missouri only)
1-800-366-8888
1-314-577-5336 TTY

MONTANA

ROCKY MOUNTAIN POISON AND DRUG CENTER
645 Bannock Street
Denver, CO 80204-4507

Emergency Number:
1-800-525-5042 (in Montana only)

NEBRASKA

POISON CONTROL CENTER
8301 Dodge Street
Omaha, NE 68114

Emergency Numbers:
1-402-390-5555
1-800-955-9119 (Nebraska only)

NEW JERSEY

NEW JERSEY POISON INFORMATION AND EDUCATION SYSTEM
Newark Beth Israel Medical Center
201 Lyons Avenue
Newark, NJ 07112

Emergency Numbers:
1-201- 923-0764
1-800-962-1253 (in New Jersey only)
1-201-926-8008 TTY

Purpose Information is available for callers about drug use, drug interaction, drug use during pregnancy and breast feeding; advice is given regarding exposures to poisonous substances both acute and chronic. Services include telephone-based treatment, counseling, coordination of emergency services, and referrals to physicians and self-help groups.

Publications
Babysitter Guide.
Lead Poisoning Prevention.
Nonpoisonous plant list.
Telephone stickers.

NEW MEXICO

NEW MEXICO POISON AND DRUG INFORMATION CENTER
University of New Mexico
Albuquerque, NM 87131

Emergency Numbers:
1-505-848-2551
1-800-432-6868 (in New Mexico only)

NEW YORK

LONG ISLAND REGIONAL POISON CONTROL CENTER
Nassau County Medical Center
2201 Hempstead Turnpike
East Meadow, NY 11554

Emergency Numbers:
1-516-542-2323, 2324, 2325

NEW YORK CITY POISON CONTROL CENTER
455 First Avenue, Room 123
New York, NY 10016

Emergency Numbers:
1-212-340-4494
1-212-POISONS

NORTH CAROLINA

MERCY HOSPITAL POISON CONTROL CENTER
2001 Vail Avenue
Charlotte, NC 28207

Emergency Numbers:
1-704-379-5827

OHIO

CENTRAL OHIO POISON CENTER
Children's Hospital
700 Children's Drive
Columbus, OH 43205

Emergency Numbers:
1-614-228-1323
1-800-682-7625 (in Ohio only)
1-614-228-2272 TTY

REGIONAL POISON CONTROL SYSTEM AND
DRUG AND POISON INFORMATION
231 Bethesda Avenue, M.L. #144
Cincinnati, OH 45267-01044

Emergency Numbers:
1-513-558-5111
1-800-872-5111 (in Ohio only)

OREGON

OREGON POISON CENTER
Oregon Health Sciences University
3181 S.W. Sam Jackson Park Road
Portland, OR 97201

Emergency Numbers:
1-503-279-8968 (local)
1-800-452-7165 (in Oregon only)

PENNSYLVANIA

DELAWARE VALLEY REGIONAL POISON CONTROL CENTER
One Children's Center
34th & Civic Center Blvd.
Philadelphia, PA 19104

Emergency Number:
1-215-386-2100

PITTSBURGH POISON CENTER
Children's Hospital of Pittsburgh
1 Children's Plaza
3705 Fifth Avenue at DeSoto Street
Pittsburgh, PA 15213

Emergency Numbers:
1-412-681-6669

RHODE ISLAND

RHODE ISLAND POISON CENTER
Rhode Island Hospital
593 Eddy Street
Providence, RI 02903

Emergency Numbers:
1-401-277-5727

TEXAS

NORTH TEXAS POISON CENTER
Parkland Hospital
5201 Harry Hints Blvd.
P.O. Box 35926
Dallas, TX 75235

Emergency Numbers:
1-214-590-5000
1-800-441-0040 (in Texas only)

TEXAS STATE POISON CENTER
The University of Texas Medical Branch
8th and Mechanic Streets
Galveston, TX 77550-2780

Emergency Numbers:
1-409-765-1420
1-713-654-1701 (in Houston)
1-512-478-4490 (in Austin)
1-800-392-8548 (in Texas only, physicians and ambulance personnel only)

UTAH

INTERMOUNTAIN REGIONAL POISON CONTROL CENTER
50 North Medical Drive; Building 528
Salt Lake City, Utah 84132

Emergency Numbers:
1-801-581-2151
1-800-456-7707 (in Utah only)

WEST VIRGINIA

WEST VIRGINIA POISON CENTER
West Virginia University Health Sciences Center/
Charleston Division
3110 MacCorkle Avenue, S.E.
Charleston, WV 25304

Emergency Numbers:
1-304-348-4211
1-800-642-3625 (in West Virginia only)

WYOMING

ROCKY MOUNTAIN POISON AND DRUG CENTER
645 Bannock Street
Denver, CO 80204-4507

Emergency Number:
1-800-442-2702 (in Wyoming only)

POISON IVY

See under Allergy.

POLIOMYELITIS (INFANTILE PARALYSIS)

An acute viral infection with a wide range of manifestation that may or may not include weakness of various muscle groups.

POLIO SURVIVORS ASSOCIATION
12720 La Reina Avenue
Downey, CA 90242

1-310-862-4508

Purpose Education, support, and advocacy for survivors of polio.

Publications

Newsletter, information relating to polio and long-term disability.

Poliomyelitis Fact Sheet, background material on polio and polio's late effects.

POLYCYSTIC KIDNEY DISEASE (PKD)

PKD affects both kidneys, enlarging them and causing symptoms, including pain, bleeding, and kidney stones. Associated problems include liver cysts and aneurysms of brain or abdomen. A high percentage of PKD patients develop kidney failure and require dialysis or transplant. PKD is an inherited condition that often remains dormant until age 30. It affects approximately 400,000 people in the United States.

NATIONAL INSTITUTE OF DIABETES AND DIGESTIVE AND KIDNEY DISEASES (NIDDKD) *1-301-499-3583*
Building 31, Room 9A04
Bethesda, MD 20892

Publications

Extracorporeal Shock-Wave Lithotripsy . . . . A Treatment for Kidney Stones, NIH Pub. No 88-859.

Prevention and Treatment of Kidney Stones, NIH Pub. No. 83-2495.

POLYCYSTIC KIDNEY RESEARCH FOUNDATION (PKRF) *1-816-421-1869*
922 Walnut, Suite 411 *1-800-PKD-CURE*
Kansas City, MO 64106

Purpose The PKRF, a nonprofit organization formed in 1982, is devoted entirely to research into the cause and cure of polycystic kidney disease. The Foundation works to educate social agencies and the public and assists patients in finding mutual support groups. There are 14 Friends groups across the United States. Referrals to physicians are not made, but patients are referred to the group coordinator.

Publications

Information packets on the disease and Foundation are mailed to each caller or written inquiry. The Foundation sells manuals, a diet book, and other publications.

POLYMYALGIA RHEUMATICA

See Arthritis, page 30.

Severe pain and stiffness in muscles without permanent weakness. Onset may be sudden or gradual; pain and stiffness may appear in the neck, shoulder, or pelvis. Morning stiffness is marked.

Write to:

ARTHRITIS FOUNDATION *1-800-283-7833*
P.O. Box 19000
Atlanta, GA 30326

PORT WINE STAIN

A birth mark, it is a purplish-red, often extensive, and sometimes partly raised area, that generally occurs singly on the face or limbs. Generally, a port wine stain persists into adult life, although it may fade slightly. Related disorders are Sturge-Weber syndrome (see page 288), Klippel-Trenaunay syndrome, blue rubber Bleb syndrome, Maffucci's syndrome, hemangiomas, and other related vascular malformations.

NATIONAL CONGENITAL PORT WINE STAIN FOUNDATION *1-212-755-3820*
125 East 63rd Street
New York, NY 10021

Purpose The Foundation is an organization formed to serve the needs of individuals and families with a member who has a port wine stain. The first goal of the foundation is to collect and disseminate information to any individual or organization concerning the symptoms, diagnosis, treatment, and prevention of congenital port wine stains. Second, the organization aims to sponsor, design, and conduct counseling and self-help programs for persons with port wine stains.

STURGE-WEBER FOUNDATION *1-303-360-7290*
P.O. Box 460931 *1-800-627-5482*
Aurora, CO 80046

Publication
Laser Treatment for Port Wine Stains, a pamphlet that discusses all aspects of treatment using the tunable dye laser.

PRADER-WILLI SYNDROME

Prader-Willi syndrome is a birth defect characterized by weak muscles, insatiable appetite, obesity if not controlled, incomplete sexual development, some degree of mental retardation or functional retardation in most cases, short stature, small hands and feet, behavior problems, and development delays.

PRADER-WILLI SYNDROME ASSOCIATION (PWSA) *1-612-926-1947*
6490 Excelsior Blvd., Suite E-102 *1-800-926-4797*
St. Louis Park, MN 55426

Purpose The PWSA serves as a national organization which acts as a clearinghouse for communication for any interested persons with any connection to the Prader-Willi syndrome. The association acts as an educational, advisory, and development headquarters furnishing information, referrals, and newsletters.

Publication
Prader-Willi Syndrome, a brochure.
List of publications is also available.

PREGNANCY

See also Adoption; Single Mothers by Choice *under* Children.

Prenatal care is vital to the health of both mother and baby. It is not enough just to see your physician regularly. You should be informed about keeping yourself in top shape with diet and exercise and avoiding substances that may harm you or the baby. You should take advantage of the educational opportunities available to make childbirth a healthy and happy experience.

AMERICAN COLLEGE OF OBSTETRICIANS AND GYNECOLOGISTS RESOURCE CENTER (ACOG) *1-202-638-5577*
409 12th Street, S.W.
Washington, D.C. 20024-2188

Purpose With a membership of more than 31,000 physicians specializing in obstetrics-gynecologic care, the ACOG serves as a strong advocate for quality health care for women, maintaining the highest standards of clinical practice and continuing education for its members; promoting patient education and stimulating patient understanding, and involvement in, medical care; and increasing awareness among its members and the public of the changing issues facing women's health care. It responds to specific questions and refers inquirers to physicians and associations.

Publications

Contraception, a pamphlet that describes how the various contraceptives work.

The Pap Test, a pamphlet that explains the procedure and its value and includes a glossary.

Patient Education, an order form for the many other educational pamphlets and books provided by the College.

Premenstrual Syndrome, a pamphlet that describes a group of physical or behavioral changes that some women go through before their menstrual periods begin.

AMERICAN LIFE LEAGUE *1-703-659-4171*
P.O. Box 1350
Stafford, VA 22554

Purpose The League, the largest pro-life, pro-family educational organization in the United States, provides library research and speakers on any of the life issues.

Publications

A.L.L About Issues, magazine format covering human interest and information.

Communique, published twice a month, it contains the latest news from the life issues, in both medical and political fields.

Resource list available with over 300 titles covering the whole range of issues.

BE HEALTHY, INC. *1-203-822-8573*
Positive Pregnancy and Parenting Fitness *1-800-433-5523*
51 Saltrock Road *Pregnancy and parenting exercise inquiries*
Baltic, CT 06330

Purpose To train qualified professionals (R.N.s, P.T.s, C.N.M.s, and aerobic and yoga teachers) to teach an early and midpregnancy fitness and informational course; postnatal fitness (mother and baby exercises) and information. Both the prenatal and the postpartum courses encourage a healthy life-style and group support. Teacher training workshops are offered.

Publications

Be Healthy Catalog for Expectant and New Parents.

Brochures on the organization.

Positive Pregnancy and Parenting Fitness Newsletter, published three times a year.

THE GLADNEY CENTER *1-800-GLADNEY*
Maternity Home and Infant Placement Center *Maternity inquiries hotline*
2300 Hemphill *1-817-922-6000*
Fort Worth, TX 76110 *Adoption inquiries*

Purpose Residential or nonresidential maternity program for young women facing unplanned pregnancy and considering the adoption option. Also provides adoption services to infertile couples and postadoption services to all members of the adoption triad. Will provide housing, if needed, medical care, counseling, education, career development, and legal and postadoption services, all at no charge to birth mother who makes an adoption plan. It will also make referrals to physicians and self-help groups.

Publication

An American Crisis, video for medical and counseling professionals with overview of teen pregnancy crisis in America and presentation of options to the crisis pregnancy.

Discover Gladney, a brochure that describes various aspects of program for birth and adoptive mothers.

Presenting Options for Crisis Pregnancy.

NATIONAL INSTITUTE OF CHILD HEALTH AND HUMAN DEVELOPMENT (NICHHD) *1-301-496-5133*
Building 31, Room 2A32
Bethesda, MD 20892

Publications

Diagnostic Ultrasound Imaging in Pregnancy.

gnancy Basics (What You Need to Know and Do to Have a Good Healthy Baby). Also available in Spanish.

Understanding Gestational Diabetes: A Practical Guide to a Healthy Pregnancy, NIH Pub. No. 89-2788.

PRO-CHOICE ABORTION HOTLINE — *1-800-772-9100*
National Abortion Foundation — *Weekdays 9:30 A.M. to 5:30 P.M. EST*
1436 U St., N.W. — *1-800-424-2280 Canadian hotline*
Washington, D.C. 20009

Purpose The Hotline provides facts about abortion, counseling, and referrals to member clinics.

PSYCHOPROPHYLAXIS IN OBSTETRICS (ASPO/LAMAZE) — *1-800-368-4404*
1840 Wilson Blvd., Suite 204
Arlington, VA 22201

PREMENSTRUAL SYNDROME (PMS)

Each month, hormones rise and fall in the bloodstream of menstruating women. The two major sex hormones, estrogen and progesterone, control various physical changes. Associated with those changes may be water retention, breast tenderness, and mood changes. These emotional changes are called PMS or premenstrual tension. They usually occur in the week before menstruation begins.

NATIONAL INSTITUTE OF CHILD HEALTH AND HUMAN DEVELOPMENT (NICHHD) — *1-301-496-5133*
Building 31, Room 2A32
Bethesda, MD 20892

Publication

Facts About Dysmenorrhea and Premenstrual Syndrome.

NATIONAL INSTITUTES OF HEALTH (NIH) — *1-301-496-2563*
Office of Clinical Center Communications
Building 10, Room 1C255
Bethesda, MD 20892

Publication
Premenstrual Syndrome: Facts and Myths.

PMS ACCESS *1-800-222-4PMS*
P.O. Box 9326
Madison, WI 53715

Purpose PMS Access provides information on premenstrual syndrome and supplies a list of support groups in caller's area.

Publications
A free information packet which contains a book called *The Odds Are Almost Even* that includes a list of symptoms, charting and ways to help PMS, and general information about Madison Pharmacy Association, the sponsor of the service. There is also a booklet listing the books and tapes offered.

PRENATAL CARE
See Pregnancy.

PROGRESSIVE SUPRANUCLEAR PALSY (PSP)
A rare disorder of late middle age manifested by loss of the use of voluntary muscles, leading to muscle rigidity with progressive crippling.

THE SOCIETY FOR PROGRESSIVE SUPRANUCLEAR PALSY, INC. *1-410-484-8771*
2904-B Marnat Road
Baltimore, MD 21209

Purpose The Society is a national, all-volunteer, nonprofit membership group of patients suffering from PSP, their family members, and caregivers. A newsletter provides nonmedical information for victims of this disease. The Society advocates increased research into progressive supranuclear palsy.

PROSTATE
See also under Aging.

The prostate is a walnut-sized gland in the pelvis. It produces fluid that helps to nourish and transport sperm. Enlargement of the prostate is a noncancerous condition of unknown cause that is increasingly common in men over the age of 50. The prostate surrounds the urethra, the tube that carries urine from the bladder through the penis. As men age, noncancerous tumors often enlarge the prostate and block the flow of urine through the urethra, leading to more frequent urination and other symptoms such as hesitancy or difficulty in starting urination.

NATIONAL INSTITUTE OF DIABETES AND DIGESTIVE AND KIDNEY DISEASES (NIDDKD) *1-301-499-3583*
Building 31, Room 9A04
Bethesda, MD 20892

Publication
Prostate Enlargement Benign Prostatic Hyperplasia, NIH Pub. No. 90-3012.

PSEUDOXANTHOMA ELASTICUM
See under Arthritis Foundation.

PSORIATIC ARTHRITIS
See under Arthritis Foundation.

PSYCHIATRIC
See American Psychiatric Association *under* Mental Health.

PSYCHOLOGICAL
See Mental Health.

PUBERTY
This is the age when children begin to develop adult sexual characteristics, capabilities and feelings. The stage usually occurs between the ages of 10 and 14 years.

NATIONAL INSTITUTE OF CHILD HEALTH AND HUMAN DEVELOPMENT (NICHHD) *1-301-496-5133*
Building 31, Room 2A32
Bethesda, MD 20892

Publication
Facts About Precocious Puberty.

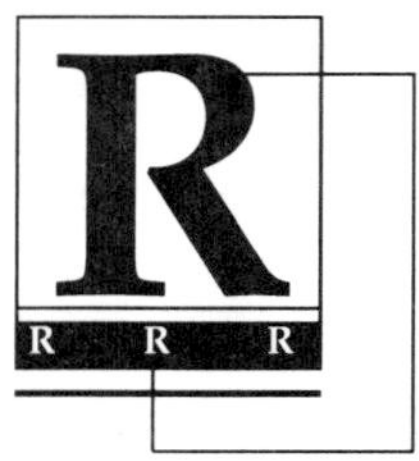

RABIES (HYDROPHOBIA)

Rabies is a potentially lethal disease caused by viruses which have an affinity for the brain and nervous tissue. The virus is transmitted to humans by the bite of an infected animal. The saliva of a rabid animal can cause the disease merely by coming in contact with abraded or scratched skin.

NATIONAL INSTITUTE OF ALLERGY AND INFECTIOUS DISEASES (NIAID) — *1-301-496-5717*
Building 31, Room 7A32
Bethesda, MD 20892

Publication
Rabies, NIH Pub. No. 83-221.

RADIATION

See also X-Ray.

Radiation is used for the diagnosis of internal conditions and the treatment of disease by either radioactivity or x-rays. Radiation therapy is mainly used to destroy cancerous growths and prevent their spread.

NATIONAL INSTITUTES OF HEALTH (NIH) — *1-301-496-2563*
Office of Clinical Center Communications
Building 10, Room 1C255
Bethesda, MD 20892

Publication
Radiation Risks and Radiation Therapy, NIH Pub. No. 83-2367.

For information on workplace safety and questions about radiation dangers, contact

FOOD AND DRUG ADMINISTRATION (FDA) — *1-301-443-4690*
Division of Consumer Affairs (HFZ-210)
Center for Devices and Radiological Health
5600 Fishers Lane
Rockville, MD 20857

NATIONAL COUNCIL ON RADIATION PROTECTION 1-301-657-2652
7910 Woodmont Ave., Suite 800
Bethesda, MD 20814

NATIONAL INSTITUTE FOR OCCUPATIONAL SAFETY AND HEALTH (NIOSH) 1-513-533-8236
Hazards Evaluations and Technical Assistance Branch (R-9)
U.S. Department of Health and Human Services
4676 Columbia Parkway
Cincinnati, OH 45226

RADON

A naturally occurring radioactive gas that cannot be seen, smelled, or tasted, radon seeps into homes from the surrounding soil through cracks and other openings in the foundation. The Environmental Protection Agency estimates that 10 percent of all homes in the United States have radon levels high enough to require corrective action. And in some areas such as Iowa, 71 percent of the homes tested had unacceptable estimates. Radon can also enter homes when it is released from well water while showering, washing clothes, and performing other household chores. Your risk from developing lung cancer from radon depends upon the average annual level of radon in your home and the amount of time you are exposed to it.

1-800-SOS-RADON
A 24-hour toll-free hotline that provides information on radon testing.

An EPA booklet, *Radon Reduction Methods: A Homeowner's Guide*, is available from your state's Radon Office.

RAPE

See under Abuse, Family Violence and Sexual Assault Institute and the Self-Help organization in your state that can refer you to a local facility.

RARE DISORDERS

Any debilitating disorder that affects less than 200,000 persons is considered rare.

NATIONAL INFORMATION CENTER FOR ORPHAN DRUGS & RARE DISEASES — *1-800-336-4797*
P.O. Box 1133
Washington, D.C. 20002

NATIONAL ORGANIZATION FOR RARE DISORDERS (NORD) — *1-203-746-6518*, *1-800-999-6673*
P.O. Box 8923
New Fairfield, CT 06812

Purpose NORD was formed in 1983 in response to the orphan drug dilemma. Known therapies which could treat some rare disorders were not being manufactured because it was unprofitable for firms to do so. NORD worked with the federal government and the pharmaceutical industry to solve this, and the Orphan Drug Act was passed. NORD monitors the Drug act to ensure that it is implemented to the fullest. In addition, NORD's programs of education, service, and research provide help and hope to people affected by these serious conditions. NORD's networking program puts individuals in touch with others who may be suffering from the same or similar illness.

Publications

Because of demand and limited funds, NORD asks for a donation, if possible, when requesting publications.

NORD brochure.

NORD literature order form.

Orphan Disease Update, a newsletter.

RAYNAUD'S PHENOMENON

See also Raynaud's Phenomenon, pages 30, 42.

A spasm of small blood vessels, usually in the hands and feet and sometimes in the nose and tongue, Raynaud's Phenomenon causes intermittent pallor or a bluish color of the skin. The attacks may last for minutes or hours. It may be due to Raynaud's disease or secondary to other conditions such as low thyroid.

NATIONAL INSTITUTES OF HEALTH (NIH)
Office of Clinical Center Communications
Building 10, Room 1C255
9000 Rockville Pike
Bethesda, MD 20892

Publication
Facts About Raynaud's Phenomenon, NIH Pub. No. 90-2263.

REFLEX SYMPATHETIC DYSTROPHY

See also Reflex Sympathetic Dystrophy Syndrome, page 30.

This condition occurs following injury to bone and soft tissue. The diagnosis depends on the association of pain with symptoms such as sweating or dizziness or atrophy of skin or bone or loss of hair.

REFLEX SYMPATHETIC DYSTROPHY ASSOCIATION (RSDA) *1-609-858-6553*
332 Haddon Ave., Suite C
Westmont, NJ 08108

Purpose The RSDA is a nonprofit professional and consumer organization founded in 1984 to support research into the cause, treatment, and cure of reflex sympathetic dystrophy syndrome, a multisymptom syndrome usually affecting one or more of the extremities, although any part of the body may be affected. The only common symptom in all patients is pain. RSDA has established the only national data bank on reflex sympathetic dystrophy to coordinate research and treatment, help organize support groups, promote awareness among health professionals, and develop educational forums and conventions.

Publications
Booklet, more extensive description of RSDS.
Brochure, a brief description of RSDS and membership form.

REHABILITATION

See also Physical Therapy.

This is a specialty in which physicians and therapists attempt to help a patient to function in a normal or near normal manner after an illness or an injury.

KESSLER INSTITUTE FOR REHABILITATION *1-201-731-3600*
Pleasant Valley Way *Ext. 369 Admissions, Ext. 304 Public Relations*
West Orange, NJ 07052 *1-800-648-0296*

Purpose With facilities in West Orange, East Orange, Saddle Brook, and Union, New Jersey, as well as an affiliate in Chester, New Jersey, Kessler Institute is the largest nonprofit rehabilitation facility in the country. Most patients are individuals who must completely reconstruct their lives due to dramatic changes which were brought on by a disabling illness or injury such as spinal cord or brain injuries, amputations, strokes, and degenerative diseases. In addition, outpatient services are provided. The goal of all Kessler programs is to assist disabled individuals in achieving a life-style that is as independent and productive as possible. Referrals are made to physicians or self-help groups when necessary upon discharge. Kessler offers several support groups, answers inquiries, provides advisory and reference services, makes referrals to other sources of information, and permits onsite use of collection.

Publications

A brochure which contains an overview of all Kessler services is available, as well as many service-specific brochures for individuals with work-related injuries, arthritis, chronic pain, and various other illnesses.

NATIONAL REHABILITATION INFORMATION CENTER (NARIC)
8455 Colesville Rd., Suite 935
Silver Spring, MD 20910

1-301-588-9284 (Voice/TDD)
1-800-34-NARIC
Fax 1-301-587-1967

Purpose NARIC is an information center on disability and rehabilitation issues and research, providing reference and referral services as well as custom database searches of the REHABDATA bibliographic database. Funded by the National Institute on Disability and Rehabilitation Research (NIDRR), NARIC collects and disseminates the results of federally funded research projects. NARIC has more than 30,000 documents on all aspects of disability and rehabilitation, including physical disabilities, psychiatric disabilities, medical rehabilitation, supported employment, independent living, assistive technology, mental retardation, special education, and law and public policy. NARIC information specialists provide individualized assistance to patrons and tailor the information provided to the needs of the user.

Publications

Most of the publications are available in large print or braille editions and cassette formats, and all are available on IBM-compatible diskette.

NARIC Quarterly, a free newsletter of disability research and resources. Each issue contains coverage of projects funded by the National Institute of Disability and Rehabilitation Research, new resources and publications available from NARIC and elsewhere, and a national calendar of disability-related conferences and events.

NARIC resource guides, designed to introduce readers to organizations, resources, and documents pertaining to a specific disability or condition. Resource guides on traumatic brain injury and spinal cord injury are available.

Rehab Brief, an NIDRR-funded publication that summarizes research findings. Each issue is devoted to a specific topic. A subject index of *Rehab Brief* is also available.

REITER'S SYNDROME

Reiter's syndrome is a arthritis associated with inflammations of the genitourinary tract, eyes, and mucous membranes as well as the joints.

ARTHRITIS FOUNDATION *1-800-283-7833*
P.O. Box 19000
Atlanta, GA 30326

Publication
Reiter's Syndrome, #4350.

RESTLESS LEG SYNDROME

A sense of uneasiness, twitching, or restlessness that occurs in the legs after going to bed, frequently leading to insomnia, which may be relieved temporarily by walking about. It is thought to be caused by inadequate circulation or as a side effect of medication.

RESTLESS LEG SYNDROME ASSOCIATION
1674 Hilcorte Dr.
Escondido, CA 92026

Purpose This small organization is an offshoot of the National Association of Rare Disorders. It is made up of victims of restless leg and their supporters. There is no charge to belong or for information. The organization refers inquiries to sources of information and to physicians specializing in this disorder. Send a stamped, self-addressed envelope when requesting information.

Publication
RLS Nightwalker, the RLSA newsletter.

RETINITIS PIGMENTOSIS (RP)

See Blindness.

A slowly progressive degeneration of the retina, the lining at the back of the eye that receives light. The layer of light-sensitive nerve cells is called rods and cones because of their shapes. The affected retinal rods produce defective night vision that may begin being a problem in childhood. Total blindness may eventually ensue.

RP FOUNDATION FIGHTING BLINDNESS *1-410-225-9400*
1401 Mount Royal Ave., 4th Floor *1-800-683-5555*
Baltimore, MD 21217-4245 *Fax 1-410-225-3936*
1-410-225-9409 TDD

Purpose Main focus of Foundation is to provide funds for research into the cause, prevention, and cure of retinitis pigmentosis and related retinal degenerations. Provides information and referral to services, support networks, and physicians specializing in the treatment of RP.

TEXAS ASSOCIATION OF RETINITIS PIGMENTOSA, INC. (TARP) *1-512-852-8515*
P.O. Box 8388
Corpus Christi, TX 78468-8388

Purpose The Association provides services for persons with retinitis pigmentosa and other progressive eye conditions. Four components render TARP a viable and highly individualized service entity unlike any other in the United States: information sharing, advocacy, referral, and emotional support. Information sharing, the major component, is a vital key to self-awareness and helps to alleviate the stress and pain experienced in the fear of "going blind." Emotionally isolated from family members and close friends, a "buddy" has provided a less intimidating situation. TARP's "Buddy Network System" supplies the linkage essential in restoring personal well-being. TARP, chartered in Texas as a nonprofit organization, has been operating since 1979 as a public awareness and educational organization.

Publications

RP Messenger, a newsletter containing information and resources on topics related to blindness and hearing impairment.

Why TARP? describes the services and retinitis pigmentosa and associated disorders.

RETT SYNDROME

Rett syndrome is a disorder which occurs only in females. It has been only recently recognized since publication of the first English language report in 1983, although first discovered by an Austrian, Dr. Andreas Rett, in 1966. Girls with the syndrome show apparent normal development from 6 to 18 months, then appear to arrest in development or regress in previously acquired skills. Among the symptoms, they may exhibit the autistic features of withdrawal and isolation in the early stages but these features improve with age. They may be retarded and spastic, and in about two-third of the girls, seizures develop. The cause of Rett syndrome is not known.

INTERNATIONAL RETT SYNDROME ASSOCIATION 1-301-248-7031
8511 Rose Marie Drive
Fort Washington, MD 20744

Purpose The aim of the Association is to support and encourage efforts to determine the cause, treatment, and cure for Rett syndrome. The Association's goal is to increase public awareness and to provide information and emotional support to families of children with Rett syndrome.

Publication
Fact sheet on Rett syndrome and order form for publications.

REYE'S SYNDROME

A disease of the brain and some abdominal organs such as the liver that primarily affects children and adolescents. The cause is unknown, but it usually follows a viral illness. It has been linked to the use of aspirin during a viral illness, but this is still controversial.

NATIONAL REYE'S SYNDROME FOUNDATION, INC. *1-419-636-2679*
426 North Lewis Street *Answering machine 24 hours*
P.O. Box 829 *1-800-233-7393*
Bryan, OH 43506

Purpose The Foundation raises and provides funds for research into the cause, cure, and treatment of Reye's syndrome. It also provides information to the general public and health professionals, offers guidance for parents of Reye's victims, and sometimes makes referrals to physicians and self-help groups.

Publications
National Reye's Syndrome Foundation, a brochure describing the foundation.

Reye's Syndrome, a brochure describing the syndrome

Videotape and slide presentation will be loaned free, except for the cost of return postage. Among them are

Reye's Syndrome: Child Killer in Disguise, a 26-minute color film available in 16mm and 1/2" VHS.

Reye's Syndrome—A Race Against Time: Overview for the General Public, a half-hour slide show.

Also will provide a list of publications sold for a few cents to cover printing costs.

RHEUMATOID ARTHRITIS

See under Arthritis, LungLine *and* Lederle Laboratories.

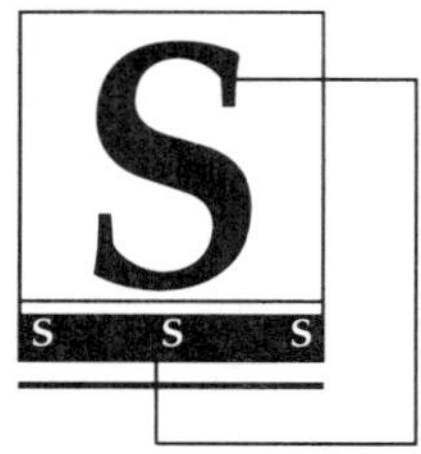

SARCOIDOSIS

See Lungline *and* Arthritis Foundation, *under* Arthritis.

SCLERODERMA

See Arthritis Foundation *and* The National Institute of Arthritis, *under* Arthritis.

SEASONS

A growing body of medical literature confirms what many people have known all along—the healing powers of sunshine. In winter, a certain percentage of people develop a condition called Seasonal Affective Depression (SAD). It's not the heat they miss, it is the light. People in the southern hemisphere develop SAD in June—when the days are shorter there. It is believed some individuals need full spectrum light to maintain their level of a brain chemical, serotonin, to avoid depression.

NATIONAL INSTITUTES OF HEALTH (NIH) *1-301-496-2563*
Office of Clinical Center Communications
Building 10, Room 1C255
Bethesda, MD 20892

Publication

Coping with the Changing Seasons, a videotape that can be borrowed.

SEIZURES

See Epilepsy.

SELF-HELP

Self-help clearinghouses refer you to find a self-help group for whatever condition you wish to contact. If none exists, many self-help clearinghouses will help you start such a group.

AMERICAN SELF-HELP CLEARING HOUSE
St. Clare's-Riverside Medical Center
Pocono Road
Denville, NJ 07834

1-800-367-6274 (in New Jersey only)
Weekdays 9 A.M. to 4 P.M. EST
1-201-625-9053 TDD
Fax 1-201-625-8848

Purpose This organization helps both laypersons and professionals to locate national and local self-help groups. It has an information line and a directory of national groups and offers consultation and registration if caller is interested in starting a new type of mutual help group or network that does not yet exist in the United States.

Publications

Provides handouts on starting a group free. Send a stamped, self-addressed business-size envelope.

Self-help Sourcebook, a directory of national and model self-help groups.

CALIFORNIA SELF-HELP CENTER
University of California—Los Angeles
2349 Franz Hall
405 Hilgard Ave.
Los Angeles, CA 90024

1-800-LINK (n California only)
Weekdays 10:00 A.M. to 6:00 P.M. PST
1-213-825-1799

Purpose A state-funded agency that offers a free information and referral service which helps thousands of people throughout the state of California to find and join self-help groups. These groups deal with problems ranging from substance abuse to bereavement to AIDS. The toll-free number provides referrals to over 4,000 self-help groups in California. If calling from outside of California, use 1-213-825-1799.

Publications

California Network of Self-help Centers, a brochure that describes the services of the California Self-Help Center and the regional centers.

Partners in Helping: Self-help Groups and Professionals Stop the Hurting, a brochure about self-help groups that deal with child abuse.

CENTER FOR SELF-HELP RIVERWOOD CENTER
P.O. Box 547
Benton Harbor, MI 49022-0547

1-800-336-0341

FULTON COUNTY SELF-HELP CLEARINGHOUSE
Clearinghouse Coordinator
113 Bleecker Street
Gloversville, NY 12078

1-518-725-4310

Purpose The Fulton County Self-Help Clearinghouse is a member of the New York State Self-Help Clearinghouse and provides information and referral pertaining to self-help/mutual aid resources available to residents of Fulton County, New York. The Clearinghouse also publishes a directory of area self-help/mutual aid groups, provides technical assistance to new and existing groups, and works to educate the community about the possibility and reality of the self-help movement.

HELPLINE *1-800-346-2211 (New York only)*
Operations Manager
29 Denison Parkway E, Suite B
Corning, New York 14830

Purpose HELPLINE is a program of a private nonprofit organization, the Institute for Human Services, designed to provide general information and referral services to Steuben County residents on a 24-hour basis by connecting them to needed services and/or helping to find answers to questions. TTY/TDD is available for those with hearing impairments. There is intake for a free countywide financial counseling program. HELPLINE works with its sponsoring program to identify unmet needs and develop services to meet them. It assists in coordinating human service programs for the county and serves as a self-help clearinghouse for Steuben County by connecting people with common concerns, helping to establish new support groups as needed, and providing technical assistance to existing groups.

MICHIGAN SELF-HELP CLEARINGHOUSE *1-517-484-7373*
Michigan Protection & Advocacy Service, Inc. *1-800-752-5858*
Clearinghouse Director
Resource Specialist
Clearinghouse Secretary
109 W. Michigan Avenue, Suite 900
Lansing, Michigan 48933

Purpose The Michigan Self-Help Clearinghouse is a statewide resource center created to promote the use of self-help/mutual aid groups by Michigan residents. It is funded by the Michigan Department of Mental Health. Because the Clearinghouse serves the entire state, it can develop supportive connections among people with similar concerns whether the need is local, regional, statewide, or national. The Clearinghouse maintains a computerized information and referral database of self-help groups throughout Michigan that is available through its toll-free number. If no group exists, the caller has the opportunity to be placed on a "seeker" list and be connected to other callers who share his or her concerns. The Clearinghouse periodically conducts surveys of self-help groups and updates existing group data. It offers phone consultation to people wanting to start groups or share their successful group experiences. Written materials on a wide range of common group problems are available. A computerized Resource Library containing self-help books, research articles, self-help group pamphlets, and handouts for which bibliographic printouts are accessible by topic area. All services are available free of charge, and there are no eligibility requirements, but because of budget cuts, the Clearinghouse would appreciate a donation to help meet operating costs.

Publications

Choosing a Self-help Group, by Toni A. Young, A.C.S.W.

The Clearinghouse Advisor on Fundraising.

Helping Ourselves, a quarterly newsletter which focuses on self-help events, making "seeker" connections, publicizing new groups in the formative stages, and encouraging the sharing of expertise among self-helpers.

Promoting Your Self-help Group, by Renee Skower.

Public Relations Strategies, by Marie Key.

Publicizing Your Self-help Group, by Faye R. Morrison, volunteer.

NORTH CAROLINA DEPARTMENT OF HUMAN RESOURCES, CARE-LINE *1-800-662-7030*
325 N. Salisbury St.
Raleigh, NC 27603

Purpose This organization offers a computerized telephone service which serves as a clearinghouse for information concerning human service programs available in all 100 counties of the state. Four incoming toll-free lines are staffed Monday through Friday from 8 A.M. to 5 P.M. A TDD is available to assist callers who are deaf or hearing impaired. Services listed include municipal, county, state, and federal government agencies; nonprofit organizations, and self-help groups. Each CARE-LINE call is handled promptly by trained staff who answer questions on programs, assess client needs, and direct clients to appropriate agencies.

Publication

Brochure that briefly describes services with hours of operation and toll-free numbers.

SELF-HELP CENTER *1-708-328-0471*
1600 Dodge Ave., Suite S-122 *1-708-328-0470*
Evanston, IL 60201

Purpose Although small and understaffed, the Center can offer a list of directories and other self-help materials for sale.

SUPPORT GROUP NETWORK AT LEXINGTON MEDICAL CENTER *1-803-791-9227*
2720 Sunset Boulevard
West Columbia, SC 29169

Purpose The Network began operation in October 1986. Its main services are to provide information and referral to mutual support groups in the Richland/Lexington County areas of South Carolina and to assist in starting new support groups where one does not exist. Seven categories of group needs have been identified: addictions/dependencies: bereavement/death, health problems; disabilities/injuries, mental health, parenting, and life situations/transitions. Hours of operation are 8:00 A.M. to 4:30 P.M., EST Monday through Friday. An answering machine records calls after hours.

WESTCHESTER SELF-HELP CLEARINGHOUSE *1-914-949-6301*
456 North Street
White Plains, NY 10605

Purpose The Westchester Clearinghouse is a central resource for information and referral to more than 250 self-help groups in Westchester County. Confidential telephone referrals are made.

OTHER SELF-HELP CLEARINGHOUSES IN THE UNITED STATES

Connecticut	*1-203-789-7645*
Iowa	*1-800-383-4777 (in Iowa)*
Kansas	*1 800-445-0116 (in Kansas); 1-316-689-3843*
Massachusetts	*1-413-545-2313*
Minnesota	*1-612-224-1133*
Missouri (Kansas City)	*1-816-561-HELP*
Nebraska	*1-402-476-9668*
New York—Brooklyn	*1-718-875-1420*
New York—Long Island	*1-516-348-3030*
North Carolina—Mecklenberg area	*1-704-331-9500*
Ohio—Dayton area	*1-513-225-3004*
Oregon—Portland area	*1-503-222-5555*
Pennsylvania—Pittsburgh area	*1-412-261-5363*
Pennsylvania—Scranton area	*1-717-961-1234*
South Carolina—Midlands area	*1-803-791-9227*
Tennessee—Knoxville area	*1-615-584-6736*
Texas	*1-512-454-3706*
Greater Washington, D.C.	*1-703-941-LINK*

SELF-HELP CLEARINGHOUSES IN CANADA

Calgary	*1-403-262-1117*
Toronto	*1-416-487-4355*
Halifax	*1-902-422-5831*
Vancouver	*1-604-731-7781*
Winnipeg	*1-204-589-5500 or 1-204-633-5955*

Publication

Initiative, national newsletter. Call 1-613-728-1865 (C.C.S.D. in Ottawa) or write

55 Parkdale Ave.
Ottawa, Ontario KIU4G1

SENILITY

See also under Aging *and* Alzheimer's.

SEX THERAPY

Anyone can claim to be a sex therapist, so it is important to get a referral from a reliable source. The first step in diagnosis is a thorough physical checkup by a physician. If your doctor cannot refer you to a sex therapist, you can call the nearest major medical center to determine if it has a sexual dysfunction clinic. If no physical problem is found and sex therapy is recommended, the organizations listed here will provide referrals to certified sex therapists in your area.

MASTERS & JOHNSON INSTITUTE *1-314-361-2377*
24 South Kingshighway
St. Louis, MO 63108

Purpose Research, treatment, and education within the broad fields of human sexuality, sexual dysfunction, communications, drugs, physical disabilities, geriatrics, ethics, contraception, psychotherapy, marriage, and homosexuality. Outpatient psychotherapy for couples and individuals with sexual dysfunctions.

Publications

List of books, journal articles and reprints.

THE NATIONAL INSTITUTE FOR THE *1-410-955-6292*
PREVENTION AND TREATMENT OF SEXUAL TRAUMA *1-410-539-1661*
104 E. Biddle Street
Baltimore, MD 21202

Purpose The Institute offers treatment for sexual offenders and treatment for victims of sexual trauma. Full psychiatric evaluations, individual counseling, group psychotherapy, treatment with the use of Dep-Provera as prescribed, and referral for inpatient hospitalization as appropriate are available.

Publications
Descriptive brochure of services and policies. Also available are articles from journals authored by the director of the clinic, Fred S. Berlin, M.D., Ph.D.

SEXAHOLICS ANONYMOUS *1-805-581-3343*
P.O. Box 300
Simi Valley, CA 93062

Purpose This organization offers a program of recovery for those who want to stop their sexually self-destructive thinking and behavior. Follows the 12-Step Fellowship Program.

Publications
Sexaholics Anonymous, a brochure.
Other literature available upon request.

SEXUAL DISORDERS CLINIC AT JOHNS HOPKINS HOSPITAL *1-410-955-6292*
Johns Hopkins Hospital *1-410-539-1661*
Meyer 4-181
600 N. Wolfe St.
Baltimore, MD 21205

Purpose The Clinic is primarily concerned with the treatment of paraphilic sexual disorders of the paraphilia such as pedophilia, exhibitionism, voyeurism, rapism, homosexual and heterosexual pedophilia, sexual sadism, hypersexuality, transvestism, and other psychosexual disorders. It will answer simple telephone inquiries without charge.

Publication
The Sexual Disorders Clinic at The Johns Hopkins Hospital, a brochure.

SURVIVORS OF INCEST ANONYMOUS, INC. (SIA) *1-410-433-2365*
P.O. Box 21817
Baltimore, MD 21222

Purpose Twelve-step, self-help recovery program for adult survivors of child sexual abuse is offered. There are no dues or fees. SIA defines incest very broadly. It makes referrals to support groups, offers pen pals for support, and provides speakers.

Publications
Send a stamped, self-addressed envelope for
Bimonthly News Bulletins.
Survivors of Incest Anonymous, a brochure that includes the 12 steps.
Survivors of Incest Anonymous: Survivors Reaching Out to Survivors, a brochure.
Survivors of Incest literature order form.

SEXUALITY

Sexuality is a great gift providing the most intimate communication possible. It can, however, also be the root of prejudice, violence, unwanted children, and deadly disease and thus heart-breaking pain. Education is vital to protect healthy sexuality.

NATIONAL INSTITUTE ON AGING (NIA) *1-301-496-1752*
Federal Building, Room 6C12
Bethesda, MD 20892

Publication

Sexuality in Later Life.

SIECUS (SEX INFORMATION AND EDUCATION COUNCIL OF THE UNITED STATES) *1-212-819-9770*
Fax 1-212-819-9776
130 West 42nd St., Suite 2500
New York, NY 10036

Purpose SIECUS affirms that sexuality is a natural part of living and advocates the right of individuals to make responsible sexual choices. SIECUS develops, collects and disseminates information and promotes education about sexuality. Has a research library and makes referral to sexual dysfunction clinics and organizations but not to individual therapists.

Publications

SIECUS: Three Decades of Commitment to Sexual Health And Education, a brochure.

SIECUS Publications Catalog, listing of materials for sale that SIECUS has available.

SEXUALLY TRANSMITTED DISEASES

Sexually transmitted diseases (STDs), also called venereal diseases, are among the most common infectious diseases in the United States. At least 20 STDs have now been identified, and they affect more than 10 million men and women each year. Although there is no sure way for a sexually active person to avoid exposure to STDs, you can reduce the risk, according to the National Institute of Allergy and Infectious Diseases, by

- Being direct and frank about asking a new sex partner whether he or she has an STD, has been exposed to one, or has any unexplained physical symptoms.
- Learning to recognize the physical signs of STDs and inspect a sex partner's body, especially the genital area, for sores, rashes, or discharges.
- Using a condom during sexual intercourse and learning to use it correctly.

Diaphragms or spermicides (particularly those containing nonoxynol-9) alone or in combination also may reduce the risk of transmission of some STDs.

AMERICAN SOCIAL HEALTH ASSOCIATION (ASHA)
P.O. Box 13827
Research Triangle Park, NC 27709

National AIDS Hotline
1-800-342-AIDS (2437) 7 days a week, 24 hours a day
1-800-344-SIDA Spanish 7 days a week, 8 A.M. to 2 A.M. EST
1-800-AIDS-TTY Hearing impaired 10 A.M. to 10 P.M. EST

National STD Hotline
1-800-227-8922 Weekdays, 8 A.M. to 11 P.M. EST

National Herpes Hotline
1-919-361-8488 Weekdays, 9 A.M. to 7 P.M. EST

Purpose ASHA is a national, nonprofit organization working for the elimination of sexually transmitted disease through its programs of education, research, and public policy. ASHA's public education program provides accurate and sensitive information in English and Spanish to those infected with STD and to those at high risk. Referrals are made to physicians or self-help groups.

Publications
Chlamydia. Also available in Spanish.
Condoms.
The Helper, a quarterly newsletter for those infected with herpes.
Herpes. Also available in Spanish.
HIV (AIDS).
HPV (Genital Warts).
HPV News, a quarterly newsletter for those infected with HPV or genital warts. Also available in Spanish.
NGU (Nongonococcal Urethritis).
PID (Pelvic Inflammatory Disease).
STD (VD).
Teens.
Women and Babies.

LEDERLE LABORATORIES *1-201-831-4692*
Public and Government Affairs
One Cyanamid Plaza
Wayne, NJ 07470

Publication

Some Questions and Answers About Chlamydia, a pamphlet on diagnosis and treatment.

NATIONAL GAY AND LESBIAN TASK FORCE (NGLTF) *1-202-332-6483*
1734 14th St., N.W. *1-202-332-6219 TTY*
Washington, D.C. 20009-4309

Purpose The 17,000-member NGLTF is the oldest national gay and lesbian civil rights advocacy organization. NGLTF lobbies, organizes, educates, and demonstrates for full gay and lesbian civil rights and equality. The Task Force is an information clearinghouse for the gay and lesbian community and the media. Since 1982, NGLTF has lobbied and testified extensively on federal AIDS policy and has helped secure passage of the Federal Hate Crimes Statistics Act, Americans with Disabilities Act, and AIDS emergency relief funding (Ryan White/CARE bill).

Publications

National Gay & Lesbian Task Force, a brochure that describes projects.

Publications Index, a listing of books and pamphlets for sale.

Task Force Report, a newsletter.

NATIONAL INSTITUTE OF ALLERGY AND INFECTIOUS DISEASES (NIAID) *1-301-496-5717*
Building 31, Room 7A32
Bethesda, MD 20892

See also Herpes.

Publication

Sexually Transmitted Diseases, NIH Pub. No. 87-909

NATIONAL LESBIAN AND GAY HEALTH FOUNDATION (NLGHF) *1-202-797-3708*
P.O. Box 65472
Washington, D.C. 20035

Purpose The Foundation focuses attention on the unique health care needs of gay men and lesbians. NLGHF works with nationwide health care professionals, the National Institutes of Health, the Centers for Disease Control, the U.S. Public Health Service, and countless state and local agencies and community organizations. The organization holds the National Lesbian and Gay Health Conference annually.

Publications

NLGHF: The National Lesbian and Gay Health Foundation, a brochure.
Publications list.

SHINGLES

Shingles (*Herpes zoster*) is the result of infection by the same virus that causes chicken pox. During an attack of chicken pox, the virus may find its way to the root of a nerve in the brain or spinal cord and hide there, often for many years, until it is reactivated. Then the virus multiplies and produces intense, knifelike pain in the nerve where it has lodged.

NATIONAL INSTITUTE OF NEUROLOGICAL DISORDERS AND STROKE (NINDS) *1-301-496-5751*
Building 31, Room 8A06
Bethesda, MD 20892

Publication

Shingles, NIH Pub. No. 82-307.

SICKLE CELL DISEASE

This is an inherited disease in which the red blood cells are shaped like sickles and contain an abnormal hemoglobin called "hemoglobin S." Symptoms include anemia and an occasional "crisis" produces an attack of pain in the bones and abdomen. Blood clots may develop in the lungs, kidney, and other organs.

HEALTH AND HUMAN SERVICES, DEPARTMENT OF; *1-301-496-6931, 6932, 6933*
PUBLIC HEALTH SERVICE; NATIONAL INSTITUTES OF HEALTH;
NATIONAL HEART, LUNG, AND BLOOD INSTITUTE;
SICKLE CELL DISEASES BRANCH
7550 Wisconsin Ave.
Bethesda, MD 20892

Purpose The Branch establishes sickle cell disease centers, supports basic and clinical research, sponsors mission-oriented research and development projects, and conducts information and education programs for professionals and the public. It also undertakes sickle cell anemia blood disease research, education, diagnosis, and counseling; answers inquiries; provides advisory, reference, literature searching, abstracting, indexing, and reproduction services; distributes information kits; lends films; and permits onsite use of reference materials.

Publications

Reports, directories, information kits, including a list of national, regional, and local groups providing sickle cell disease services; a list of screening and education clinics, brochures; and reprints. A publications list is available. Services are free and available to anyone.

NATIONAL ASSOCIATION FOR SICKLE CELL DISEASE *1-800-421-8453*
4221 Wilshire Blvd., Suite 360
Los Angeles, CA 90010-3505

NATIONAL INSTITUTES OF HEALTH (NIH) *1-301-496-2563*
Office of Clinical Center Communications
Building 10, Room 1C255
Bethesda, MD 20892

Publication

Sickle Cell Anemia, NIH Pub. No. 90-3058.

SINUSITIS

The sinuses are holes in your head, specifically the air spaces in the bones behind your nose. Sinusitis is an inflammation of the mucous membranes of the sinuses; it is caused by a bacterial or viral infection.

AMERICAN ACADEMY OF OTOLARYNGOLOGY
HEAD AND NECK SURGERY (AAOHNS)
One Prince Street
Alexandria, VA 22314

Publication

SINUS, Pain and Pressure.

OWEN ALLERGY AND SINUS CENTER *615-327-3291*
1801 Church St.
Nashville, TN 37203

Publication
Endoscopic Sinus Surgery Procedures.

SJOGREN'S SYNDROME

See Arthritis Foundation, *under* Arthritis.

SKIN CANCER

Skin cancer afflicts more people than any other form of cancer; over 600,000 new cases will be diagnosed in the United States this year. Yet with early detection and effective treatment, virtually all skin cancers are curable. Learning how to examine your own skin from head to toe is the best way to spot skin cancer in its earliest, most treatable stages.

SKIN CANCER FOUNDATION — *1-212-725-5176*
245 Fifth Ave., Suite 2402 — *Fax 1-212-725-5751*
New York, NY 10016

Purpose A nonprofit foundation, it is the only national organization concerned solely with the world's most prevalent malignancy—cancers of the skin. The Foundation conducts public and medical education programs and provides support for research to help reduce the incidence, morbidity, and mortality of skin cancer.

Publications
Public Information Catalog.

SKIN PROBLEMS

The skin is one of the largest organs of the body. It is a supple, elastic tissue that prevents the loss of moisture and heat. It not only protects you from the environment but tells you about what is going on outside yourself. It senses, for example, and then helps regulate temperature. Its pain sensors warn of potential damage from sharp or hot things. Because it is so exposed to external and internal environments, a lot can go wrong with it.

AMERICAN ACADEMY OF DERMATOLOGY — *1-708-869-3954*
P.O. Box 3116 — *Fax 1-708-869-4382*
Evanston, IL 60204-3116

Purpose The Academy offers continuing medical education for dermatologists, provides 35 pamphlets for consumer education, and refers to board-certified dermatologists anywhere in the world and to self-help groups.

Publications

Thirty-five pamphlets about skin problems, including acne and skin cancers.

AMERICAN SOCIETY FOR DERMATOLOGIC SURGERY *1-708-869-3954*
1567 Maple Avenue *1-800-441-2737*
P.O. Box 3116
Evanston, IL 60204-3116

Purpose Dermatologic surgeons are physicians who have completed an internship and three additional years of specialized training in the medical and surgical treatment of skin disorders. In addition to providing education and training to its 2,200 members, the organization provides information such as fact sheets and pamphlets on various skin conditions and treatments in dermatologic surgery to laypersons. Consumers will also receive a referral list of dermatologic surgeons who specialize in particular procedures and conditions who are located in the consumer's geographic area.

Publications

Brochures on dermatologic surgery and the use of lasers in dermatologic surgery and chemical peel.

Fact Sheets

Acne Scarring.

Aging and Sun-Damaged Skin: Chemical Peel, Dermabrasion, and Soft-Tissue Augmentation.

Aging Eyelids.

Genital Warts.

Hair Loss and Transplantation.

Liposuction and Micro-lipoinjection.

Liver Spots and Aging Hands.

Retinoids.

Skin Cancer.

Tattoo Removal.

Treatment for Spider and Varicose Veins.

SCHERING-PLOUGH CORPORATION/KEY PHARMACEUTICALS *1-908-298-4000*
2000 Galloping Hill Road
Kenilworth, NJ 07033

Publications

Bacterial Skin Infections.

Contact and Atopic Dermatitis.

Herpes Zoster (Shingles).

Lice and Scabies.

Psoriasis.

Skin Cancer.

Vaginitis: A Very Common Condition.

Warts and Moles.

SLEEP DISORDERS

An estimated 30 million Americans cannot achieve continuous sleep at night. Their sleep is fragmented and disrupted by sleep disorders, and sometimes they cannot sleep at all. Other sleep problems include

- *Narcolepsy*, which causes a person to suddenly fall asleep during the day
- *Sleep apnea syndrome*, which affects an estimated 20 million Americans and causes them to be unable to maintain breathing and normal oxygen levels during sleep
- *Stroke and epilepsy*, which occur more often during sleep than at other times
- *Sudden infant death syndrome*, which occurs when the immature sleeping brain, for as yet unproven reasons, cannot reliably maintain the life support system

NATIONAL INSTITUTES OF HEALTH (NIH) *1-301-496-2563*
Office of Clinical Center Communications
Building 10, Room 1C255
Bethesda, MD 20892

Publication

Sleep and Its Disorders, a videotape that can be borrowed.

NATIONAL SLEEP FOUNDATION *1-310-288-0466*
122 South Robertson Blvd., Suite 201 *Fax 1-310-288-0570*
Los Angeles, CA 90048

Purpose The National Sleep Foundation's mission is to improve the quality of life for millions of Americans who suffer from sleep disorders and to prevent the catastrophic accidents that are related to poor or disordered sleep. These goals are carried out through support of research, education, and the dissemination of information. The Foundation furnishes information on all aspects of sleep and its disorders.

Publications

Don't Take Sleep Problems Lying Down, gives a general overview of sleep and sleep disorders, providing insight into how to help your doctor understand the type of problem affecting your sleep.

Roster of Accredited Centers and Laboratories, regional listings of sleep disorders centers and laboratories that have complied with the American Sleep Disorders Association's standards of practice in sleep medicine.

Sleep Apnea, outlines the symptoms, causes, evaluation, and treatment of the three types of sleep apnea, courtesy of the American Sleep Disorders Association.

Sleep Problems in Children, describes both normal and disordered sleep in children through the age of 20 years, courtesy of the American Sleep Disorders Association.

Sleep as We Grow Older, discusses common problems of sleep for the elderly and offers guidelines to help individuals sleep well and feel alert during the day.

When You Can't Sleep: The ABCs of ZZZs, an insomnia quiz booklet which identifies the types of insomnia, and some of the causes and gives information on good sleep habits.

SMELL AND TASTE DISORDERS

More than 200,000 persons visit a physician for a smell or taste problem each year. Many more smell and taste disturbances go unreported.

AMERICAN ACADEMY OF OTOLARYNGOLOGY HEAD AND NECK SURGERY (AAOHNS)
One Prince Street
Alexandria, VA 22314

1-703-836-4444
Fax 1-703-683-5100

Publication

Send a stamped, self-addressed envelope for *Smell & Taste Disorders*.

NATIONAL INSTITUTE ON DEAFNESS AND OTHER COMMUNICATION DISORDERS (NIDOCD)
Clearing House
P.O. Box 37777
Washington, D.C. 20013-7777

1-301-496-7243
1-301-402-0252 TDD
Fax 1-301-402-0018

Publication

Smell and Taste Disorders, a booklet that describes current research and the importance of obtaining a proper diagnosis.

SMOKING

Based on a survey by the Surgeon General, an estimated 91.1 million adults in the United States have been smokers, and 49.4 million are current smokers. An estimated 434,175 premature deaths in the United States are attributed to cigarette smoking. In the United States, according to the Centers for Disease Control, the overall average age at which smokers began smoking cigarettes regularly decreased from 19.7 years to 17.4 years. Current smokers include 30.8 percent of all men and 25.7 percent of all women.

AMERICAN ACADEMY OF OTOLARYNGOLOGY HEAD AND NECK SURGERY (AAOHNS)
1-703-836-4444
Fax 1-703-683-5100
One Prince Street
Alexandria, VA 22314

Publication
Send a stamped, self-addressed envelope for
Smokeless Tobacco.

NATIONAL HEART, LUNG, AND BLOOD INSTITUTE (NHLBI)
1-301-496-4236
Building 31, Room 4A21
Bethesda, MD 20892

Publications
Quit to Win, poster.
Smoking and Chronic Obstructive Lung Disease (NHLBI Facts About), NIH Pub. No. 88-2887.

NATIONAL INSTITUTE ON AGING (NIA)
1-301-496-1752
Federal Building, Room 6C12
Bethesda, MD 20892

Publication
Smoking: It's Never Too Late to Stop.

OFFICE ON SMOKING AND HEALTH
1-301-443-1690
Technical Information Center
Park Building, Room 1-16
5600 Fishers Lane
Rockville, MD 20857

Purpose The Office on Smoking and Health offers bibliographic and reference services to researchers through its Technical Information Center (TIC), formerly called the National Clearinghouse for Smoking and Health. The TIC publishes and distributes a number of titles in the field of smoking and health and possesses computer capability, through its Automated Search and Retrieval System, to generate comprehensive bibliographic printouts on topics of current interest in smoking and health. In addition to the bibliographic services offered, the Office has an Epidemiology Branch for the collection and analysis of numeric data sets, primarily taken from national probability surveys sponsored within the Department, which contain significant tobacco use information. This section also designs and conducts national surveys on smoking behavior, attitudes, knowledge, and beliefs among adults and teenagers on a periodic basis and works with other individuals and organizations that are interested in incorporating smoking behavior as part of their survey research activities. Visitors may use the TIC collection weekdays from 8:30 A.M. to 5:00 P.M.. Advance arrangements for visits are suggested. Reference services are also provided by telephone. Copies of reference items can be provided only in single copies, and only in cases where material cannot be obtained from other sources.

SEVENTH-DAY ADVENTISTS COMMUNITY HEALTH SERVICES
P.O. Box 1029
Manhasset, NY 11030

Publication

You Can Stop Smoking, hints about breaking the habit. Also available in Spanish.

SNORING

See also Sleep

Some 45 percent of normal adults snore at least occasionally and 25 percent are habitual snorers. Problem snoring is more frequent in males and overweight persons, and it usually grows worse with age. More than 300 devices are registered in the U.S. Patent and Trademark Office as cures for snoring.

AMERICAN ACADEMY OF OTOLARYNGOLOGY
HEAD AND NECK SURGERY (AAOHNS)
One Prince Street
Alexandria, VA 22314

1-703-836-4444
Fax 1-703-683-5100

Publication

Send a stamped, self-addressed envelope for
Snoring—Not Funny, Not Hopeless.

SPEECH DISORDERS

Fourteen million persons in the United States experience speech or language problems.

AMERICAN SPEECH-LANGUAGE HEARING ASSOCIATION *1-301-897-5700*
10801 Rockville Pike *1-800-638-8255*
Rockville, MD 20852

Purpose This organization is a professional and scientific association of speech-language pathologists and audiologists, the professionals who treat communication disorders. Through toll-free consumer Helpline, the Association provides information about speech and hearing disorders and refers callers to speech-language pathologists and audiologists in the requestor's area. The purposes of the Association are to encourage basic scientific study of the processes of individual human communication, with special reference to speech, hearing, and language; to promote investigation of disorders of human communication and to foster improvements of clinical procedures for such disorders; to stimulate exchange of information among persons and organizations thus engaged; and to disseminate information about communication disorders to the general public, physicians, and educators. Members of the Association are interested in the nature, processes, and disorders of speech, hearing, and language, including voice disorders, aphasia, cerebral palsy, cleft palate, delayed speech, laryngectomy, and stuttering; anatomy and physiology; auditory skills and training; psychoacoustics; audiometry; auditory feedback; hearing aids; phonetics; semantics; and therapeutic techniques for speech and hearing disorders.

Publications

The following brochures are available:

American Speech-Language-Hearing Association Answers Questions About Adult Aphasia.

American Speech-Language-Hearing Association Answers Questions About Articulation Problems.

American Speech-Language-Hearing Association Answers Questions About Assistive Listening Devices.

American Speech-Language-Hearing Association Answers Questions About Child Language.

American Speech-Language-Hearing Association Answers Questions About Otitis Media.

American Speech-Language-Hearing Association Answers Questions About Otitis Medica, Hearing, and Language Development.

American Speech-Language-Hearing Association Answers Questions About Stuttering.

American Speech-Language-Hearing Association Answers Questions About Tinnitus.

American Speech-Language-Hearing Association Answers Questions About Voice Problems.
Communication Disorders And Aging.
Do Your Health Benefits Cover Audiology and Speech-Language Pathology Services?
Hearing Impairment and the Audiologist.
How Does Your Child Hear and Talk? Also available in Spanish.
Noise in Your Workplace.
Recognizing Communication Disorders.
Speech and Language Disorders and the Speech-Language Pathologist.
The Speech-Language Pathologist in the Schools.

NATIONAL INSTITUTE ON DEAFNESS AND OTHER COMMUNICATION DISORDERS (NIDOCD) *1-301-496-7243*
Building 31, Room 1B62
Bethesda, MD 20892

Publications

Developmental Speech and Language Disorders, NIH Pub. No. 88-2757, a 35-page booklet on the stages of development of children's speech and language.

Stuttering, NIH Pub. No. 81-2250, describes famous stutterers, new research, and treatments for stuttering.

NATIONAL INSTITUTES OF HEALTH (NIH) *1-301-496-2563*
Office of Clinical Center Communications
Building 10, Room 1C255
Bethesda, MD 20892

Publication

Speech and Language Disorders.

SPINA BIFIDA

In spina bifida, part of the bony spine that helps protect the spinal cord fails to develop properly. The nerves of the spinal cord in that area are exposed and unprotected and may also be defective.

NATIONAL INSTITUTE OF NEUROLOGICAL DISORDERS AND STROKE (NINDS) *1-301-496-5751*
Building 31, Room 8A06
Bethesda, MD 20892

Publication

Spina Bifida, NIH Pub. No. 85-309.

SPINA BIFIDA ASSOCIATION OF AMERICA (SBAA) *1-301-770-7222, 7223*
1700 Rockville Pike, Suite 250 *1-800-621-3141*
Rockville, MD 20852-1654

Purpose SBAA helps fund research into the cause of spina bifida, works to improve medical devices and treatment facilities for this birth defect, and encourages the training of professionals and others dealing with the care and treatment of afflicted persons. It has a network of chapters across the United States and provides leadership training for chapters in the form of workshops. Adoption information referral is offered for those looking for an option. The Association answers inquiries on spina bifida, neurological disorders, hydrocephalus, and genetic counseling; provides information on research in progress and a list of resources offering financial and other types of support to families; distributes publications; conducts national conference with seminars on scientific, social, medical, and education programs; and makes referrals to other sources of information.

Publications

Single copies of the following are free.
The Baby Doe Law, by Jack Bierig, Esq.
The Chiari Malformation, by W. Jerry Oakes, M.D.
CIC-The Law, by J. Glucksman, Esq.
Genetics, by Lowell Sever, Ph. D.
Hip Stability & Ambulation, by Richard Lindseth, M.D.
Kidney Care, by Elizabeth Jackson, M.D.
Social Aspects of Spina Bifida, by Rosalyn Darling, Ph.D.
Spina Bifida Association of America Publications & Audio Visual Materials, a publications list.
Tethered Cord, by Joan L. Venes, M.D.
Urological Care, by William Kaplan, M.D.

SPINAL CORD INJURIES

More than 250,000 Americans are paralyzed as the result of injury and disease to the spinal cord. Each year, another 12,000 people, mostly teenage males, sustain a spinal cord injury primarily as a result of motor vehicle and related accidents or crimes of violence. *Paraplegia* involves paralysis of the legs and lower parts of the body. *Quadriplegia* denotes paralysis affecting the level below the neck and chest area involving both the arms and legs.

NATIONAL INSTITUTE OF NEUROLOGICAL DISORDERS AND STROKE (NINDS) *1-301-496-5751*
Building 31, Room 8A06
Bethesda, MD 20892

Publication
Spinal Cord Injury, NIH Pub. No. 81-160.

NATIONAL SPINAL CORD INJURY ASSOCIATION (NSCIA) *1-800-962-9629*
600 W. Cummings Park, Suite 2000
Woburn, MA 01801

Purpose The Association is a private nonprofit organization established by the Paralyzed Veterans of America in 1948 as a response to the civilian medical and social problems that resulted from injury to the spinal cord. The NSCIA has more than 60 chapters and support groups through the country dedicated to its original purpose: care, cure, and coping. The NSCIA has a resource center which responds to any questions pertaining to spinal cord injury or paralysis. The organization also offers prevention education and advocacy on accessibility and transportation issues and other rights of people with disabilities.

Publications
Fact Sheets.
Options: Spinal Cord Injury & The Future.
SCI Life.
Spinal Network.

SPINAL MUSCULAR ATROPHY (WERDNIG-HOFFMANN SYNDROME)

An inherited syndrome, this is a disease of nerves that control motor functions including swallowing. There are two forms. Type I is severe and children who suffer from it are never able to lift their heads or accomplish normal physical milestones. Those with Type II may sit up unsupported and may be able to stand.

FAMILIES OF SMA (SPINAL MUSCULAR ATROPHY) *1-708-432-5551*
P.O. Box 1465
Highland Park, IL 60035

Purpose Founded by a group of parents of children with SMA, the organization works to raise money to distribute educational materials, provide patient services and support research, that will lead to prenatal testing, treatment, and cure. It fosters family networking and equipment exchange, and will make referrals to self-help groups and physicians treating the condition.

Publications

Direction, a quarterly newsletter with information regarding research and general help in all aspects of coping daily with handicapped family members.

Understanding SMA, a brochure about the condition and the organization.

SPORTS MEDICINE

Athletes and others who pursue vigorous exercise often injure muscles, ligaments, bones or joints. Physicians and therapists who specialize in sports medicine not only provide therapy for such injuries but try to prevent them from occurring.

AEROBICS AND FITNESS FOUNDATION OF AMERICA (AFFA) *1-800-BE FIT 86*
15250 Ventura Blvd., Suite 310
Sherman Oaks, CA 91403

Purpose AFFA is a nonprofit organization committed to promoting, teaching, and researching safe and effective ways to achieve fitness through aerobic exercise. AFFA also promotes fitness to the nation's youth as a positive alternative to substance abuse through SUPERCLASS events, which are hosted by health clubs. The SUPERCLASS events teach aerobics to teens in drug rehabilitation programs.

Publication

Footnotes, information cards that provide educational facts on health and exercise.

ALLERGY INFORMATION CENTER AND HOTLINE *1-800-727-5400*

Publication

How to Be a Good Sport . . . With Allergies, lists sports from bowling to rock scrambling according to their allergy-provoking potential and provides tips about how you can enjoy allergy-free workouts.

AMERICAN RUNNING AND FITNESS ASSOCIATION (AR&FA) *1-301-897-0197*
9310 Old Georgetown Road *1-800-776-ARFA*
Bethesda, MD 20814

Purpose Founded in 1968 as the National Jogging Association, this organization provides information and support programs for people interested in exercise and promotes running as a practical way of achieving physical fitness. The AR&FA offers its members information, literature, discounts on exercise equipment, and medical advice on jogging-related problems. The AR&FA challenge program aids self-motivation by encouraging runners to compete against themselves. Advice is given on how to promote running programs on the local level. It refers callers to sports medicine professionals and to local speakers.

Publications

AR&FA Publications Guide.

Members can obtain four free brochures from the FitTip Series on exercise programs, injury prevention, stretching, safety, and training by sending a stamped, self-addressed, business-size envelope.

Running and Fitness, a monthly newsletter for members reporting on the latest in sports medicine research, training tips, nutrition, and other information.

NATIONAL COLLEGIATE ATHLETIC ASSOCIATION (NCAA) *1-913-339-1906*
Sciences Division
6201 College Boulevard
Overland Park, Kansas 66211-2422

Purpose The NCAA, founded in 1906, serves as the national association for collegiate athletics. As a voluntary association of more than 900 institutions, the NCAA administers college athletics programs and rules on issues pertaining to the administration of intercollegiate athletics. Services include sponsorship of athletic championships, scholarships for college athletes to pursue graduate studies, approval and publication of rules for collegiate athletics, research on related problems and issues, compilation of statistics, promotion of events, and group insurance programs. The NCAA is also involved in medicine and safety activities. NCAA publications include position statements on such issues as safety and medicine, as well as rules of play and statistics. Provides drug education materials and programs to grade school, high school, and collegiate student-athletes.

Publications

Aggregate Drug-Testing Results, 1986 Through 1991.

Annual Survey of Catastrophic Football Injuries. 1991

Alcohol: Choices and Guidelines for College Students.

Drugs and the Athlete . . . A Losing Combination.

Drug education posters (set of three).

Injury Surveillance System Data.

Legal Implications of Mandatory Drug Testing: The Final Report of the Center for Law and Sports, June 7, 1985.

National Center of Catastrophic Injury Research.

NCAA Drug-Education and Drug-Testing Survey.

NCAA Sciences Handbook, 1992 Edition.

NCAA Sciences Newsletter.

1991–92 NCAA Drug Testing/Drug Education Programs.
1991–92 NCAA Drug-Testing Site Coordinator Manual.
Replication of the National Study of Substance Use and Abuse Habits of College Student-Athletes, October 1989.
Report of the National Consensus Meeting on Anabolic/Androgenic Steroids, July 30-31, 1989.

PRESIDENT'S COUNCIL ON PHYSICAL FITNESS AND SPORTS (PCPFS) *1-202-272-3430*
Director of Information
450 5th Street, N.W., Suite 7103
Washington, D.C. 20001

Purpose The President's Council on Physical Fitness and Sports is an outgrowth of the President's Council on Youth Fitness, established in 1956. It conducts a public service advertising program, prepares educational materials, and cooperates with governmental and private groups to promote the development of physical fitness leadership, facilities, and programs. The PCPFS also works with schools, clubs, recreation agencies, and major employers on program design and implementation; advises federal agencies on the conduct of fitness-related programs; and offers a variety of testing, recognition, and incentive programs for individuals, institutions, and organizations.

UNDERSEA & HYPERBARIC MEDICAL SOCIETY *1-301-571-1818*
9650 Rockville Pike *1-301-571-1821 Librarian*
Bethesda, MD 20814

Purpose The Undersea Medical Society, founded in 1967, seeks to advance undersea medicine and facilitate scientific communication among researchers dedicated to the safe exploration of the oceans and the use of oxygen under pressure (hyperbaric) to treat divers suffering from the bends. A scientific forum is provided through publications, annual meetings, workshops, symposia, and continuing education programs. Other services include responses to inquiries, a reference library, and an information retrieval system. The Society database provides indexed entries for more than 17,000 documents such as monographs, journal articles, and technical reports. Physician referrals are made.

STROKE

More than 500,000 Americans a year, most of them over the age of 65, suffer strokes. Many are left with language and mobility problems and become dependent on other family members for their daily needs. For suggestions on how to care for a relative recovering from stroke, including information on therapies, finances, and coping with family, write to or call the following:

AMERICAN HEART ASSOCIATION 1-214-373-6300
7272 Greenville Ave.
Dallas, TX 75231-4596

Purpose The Association is a national voluntary health agency dedicated to the reduction of premature death or disability from cardiovascular diseases and stroke. This is accomplished through research support, medical education, public education, and community demonstration programs. The organization is interested in all aspects of cardiology and cardiovascular diseases; blood, cerebral, and kidney diseases in relation to the cardiovascular system; congenital heart disease; surgery; and prevention and control of heart disease and stroke.

NATIONAL INSTITUTE OF NEUROLOGICAL DISORDERS AND STROKE (NINDS) 1-301-496-5751
Building 31, Room 8A06
Bethesda, MD 20892

Publication
Stroke, NIH Pub. No. 83-2222.

NATIONAL INSTITUTES OF HEALTH (NIH) 1-301-496-2563
Office of Clinical Center Communications
Building 10, Room 1C255
Bethesda, MD 20892

Publication
Stroke Update, NIH Pub. No. 88-2989.

NATIONAL STROKE ASSOCIATION (NGA) 1-303-762-9922
300 E. Hampden Avenue, Suite 300 1-800-STROKES
Englewood, CO 80110-2654

Purpose NSA is a nonprofit organization, incorporated in 1984, dedicated to educating stroke survivors, families, health professionals, and the general public about stroke. It seeks to reduce the incidence and effects of stroke (CVA) through activities related to prevention, medical care, rehabilitation, and resocialization. NSA develops and distributes educational materials and a newsletter, operates a national clearinghouse for information and referral, and sponsors research fellowships and symposia on stroke. Referrals to self-help groups are made; referrals to physicians are done on a limited basis.

Publications

Be Stroke Smart Adaptive Resources, a guide to manufacturers and products (single copy free).

Be Stroke Smart National Stroke Association Newsletter.

Professional & Patient, catalog of educational materials.

STURGE-WEBER SYNDROME (SWS)

In this syndrome, children are born with red skin tumors that follow the trigeminal nerve in the face and that may cause calcifications in the brain and glaucoma.

STURGE-WEBER FOUNDATION *1-202-360-7290*
P.O. Box 460931 *1-800-627-5482*
Aurora, CO 80015

Purpose This nonprofit organization for parents, professionals, and others concerned with Sturge-Weber syndrome facilitates and funds research on SWS; disseminates information on SWS; acts as a support group for all interested parties; and refers inquirers to physicians and self-help groups.

Publications

Glaucoma—What Is It? a brochure which addresses glaucoma as it relates to SWS. It is written in layperson's terms and is suitable for parents and teachers.

Laser-Treatment for Port Wine Stains, a pamphlet which discusses all aspects of treatment using the tunable dye laser.

Laymen's Guide, a guide defining medical terminology related to SWS in layperson's terms.

A Rainbow of Hope for Parents, a publication for parents of those diagnosed with SWS. It helps with the emotions parents feel when coping with SWS.

Sturge-Weber Syndrome, a brochure with a brief overview of the syndrome. It also informs the reader about SWF's activities and goals.

SWF Newsletter, published quarterly and available with a donation.

STUTTERING

See also Stuttering *under* Speech

Stuttering is a disorder usually beginning in childhood, characterized by intense anxiety about the efficiency of oral communications, and by hesitation, repetitions, and prolongations of sounds and syllables. There are interjections, broken words, and words produced with excess tension.

HEALTH AND HUMAN SERVICES, DEPARTMENT OF; PUBLIC HEALTH SERVICE; NATIONAL INSTITUTES OF HEALTH; NATIONAL INSTITUTE OF NEUROLOGICAL AND STROKE; OFFICE OF SCIENTIFIC AND HEALTH REPORTS
P.O. Box 5801
Bethesda, MD 20824
1-301-496-5751
1-800-352-9424

Purpose This agency engages in research and training relating to the causes, prevention, diagnosis, and treatment of neurological and communicative disorders. Data banks on the Institute's research and training grants and awards and on perinatal research are accessible. In reply to some inquiries, referral is made to other organizations and individuals.

Publications
A list of publications is available. Pamphlets and other publications are distributed free in response to public inquiries received through correspondence or by telephone.

NATIONAL STUTTERING PROJECT (NSP)
2151 Irving St., Room 208
San Francisco, CA 94122
1-415-566-5324
Fax 1-415-664-3721

Purpose A nonprofit self-help organization, NSP offers information on stuttering to people with speech difficulties and the general public and acts as a referral service for those seeking professional assistance. Over 100 support groups, monthly newsletter, brochures, books, and public awareness programs are available. Information and materials are provided on stuttering; referral information to speech pathologists and self-help groups is available.

Publications
Publications list. Charges for publications.

SUDDEN INFANT DEATH SYNDROME (SIDS)

See also Bereavement.

A medical puzzle, sudden infant death occurs when an apparently healthy baby is laid down to sleep and some time later dies. In nearly all cases, no explanation for the death is discovered. Research has shown that the risk of crib death is higher in the winter and may be related to the immaturity of the part of the brain that controls breathing. There have been many other explanations, but as yet, the cause or causes are not known.

NATIONAL SUDDEN INFANT DEATH SYNDROME CLEARINGHOUSE *1-301-459-3388*
8200 Professional Place, Suite 104,
Landover, MD 20785

Purpose The U.S. Public Health Service's Bureau of Health Care Delivery and Assistance's SIDS Program established the Clearinghouse to provide information and educational materials on SIDS, including theories of causation, epidemiology, identification of high-risk infants, the grieving process, counseling methods, siblings' response to SIDS, and research findings; apnea; death; and dying. The Clearinghouse, which is operated by The Circle, 8294-C Old Courthouse Rd., Vienna, VA 22180, maintains a computerized database of 700 articles, standard reference materials, and classics in the field; has a core library; answers inquiries; distributes publications; makes referrals to other sources of information; provides database searches and information on research in progress; and permits onsite use of collections. Services are free and available to anyone.

Publications
The Information Exchange, a quarterly newsletter.
Fact sheets, directories, research summaries, bibliographies, reprints.

SUICIDE

Suicide rates for adolescents 15–19 years old have quadrupled from 2.7 per 100,000 in 1950 to 11.3 in 1988. Attempted suicide is a potentially lethal health event, a risk factor for future completed suicide, and a potential indicator of other health problems such as substance abuse, depression, or adjustment and stress reactions.

AMERICAN ASSOCIATION OF SUICIDOLOGY *1-303-692-0985*
2459 S. Ash
Denver, CO 80222

Purpose This clearinghouse for information on suicide, refers callers to suicide prevention and crisis intervention centers and support groups for survivors of suicide (those who have lost a loved one to suicide), and provides educational materials and educational programs.

Publications
A variety of suicide prevention pamphlets and a resource list for survivors of those who have committed suicide.

HEMLOCK SOCIETY *1-503-342-5748*
P.O. Box 11830 *1-800-247-7421*
Eugene, OR 97440

Purpose This educational nonprofit society addresses voluntary euthanasia for the terminally ill and provides education and research. Physicians referrals are *not* made. Referrals are made to hospice and suicide prevention centers. The Society answers inquiries, provides reference services, conducts seminars and workshops, and distributes publications. Services are free, except for publications, and are available to anyone. Information is provided within legal limits; that is, no counseling is provided.

Publications

Hemlock Catalog lists publications, pins, buttons, bumper stickers, will forms, and other information on the Society and its philosophy.

SURGERY

See Plastic Surgery *and* Otolaryngology.

SYRINGOMYELIA

Syringomyelia is characterized by a fluid-filled cavity within the spinal cord or brainstem. About half the lesions are present at birth, but for unknown reasons they often expand during the teens or young adult years. The remainder arise in association with tumors.

AMERICAN SYRINGOMYELIA ALLIANCE PROJECT, INC. (ASAP) *1-903-757-7456*
P.O. Box 1586 *Fax 1-903-757-7456*
Longview, TX 75606-1586

Purpose ASAP acts as a clearinghouse of information on syringomyelia, promotes networking programs for victims, and supports research.

Publications

Bimonthly newsletter.
Malformations by physicians in the field.
Miscellaneous articles on syringomyelia and Arnold Chiari Syndrome.
Syringomyelia brochure.

SYSTEMIC LUPUS ERYTHEMATOSUS

See also pages 19, 30, 170, 185, 186, 187, and 211.

Lupus erythematosus is a chronic disorder of the immune system that causes inflammation of various parts of the body. People with lupus have immune system abnormalities. For most people lupus is a mild disease affecting only a few body organs; for others, it may cause serious and even life-threatening problems. Approximately 500,000 people in the United States suffer from systemic lupus. Among the telltale symptoms are

- A rash over the bridge of the nose
- Flushing of the cheeks or disclike rashes that appear on the face, neck, scalp, and other areas of the skin exposed to sunlight

S.L.E. FOUNDATION, INC. *1-212-685-4118*
149 Madison Ave., Suite 608 *1-212-606-1952*
New York, NY 10016

Lupus Line offered by Hospital for Special Surgery in Cooperation with The S.L.E. Foundation, Inc., provides free counseling services staffed by trained volunteers who have lupus.

Purpose A nonprofit organization, the S.L.E. (Systemic Lupus Erythematosus) Foundation, Inc., provides information and referral services, counseling, and support services to patients and loved ones and raises money to fund research into the disease. The Foundation supplies literature on a variety of lupus-related issues to anyone who requests it. In addition, the foundation offers a referral service to knowledgeable lupus specialists.

Publications
Books and Other Items Available, a brochure with order list.

Reprints of various articles on the subject.

What Is Lupus? a brochure describing the symptoms and treatment of the disease.

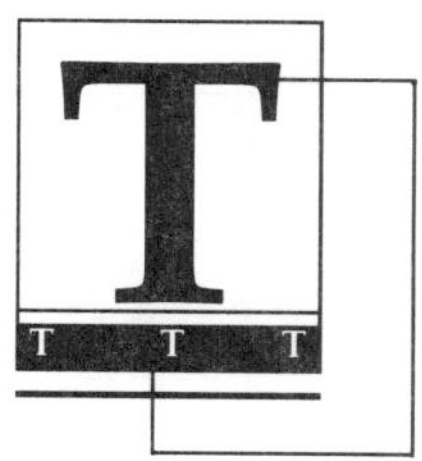

TASTE DISORDERS

Taste deficits for sweet, sour, bitter, and salty substances present serious problems because they can destroy the motivation to consume nutrients. Taste deficits may also lead to unhealthy dietary habits such as excess salt consumption.

NATIONAL INSTITUTE ON DEAFNESS AND OTHER COMMUNICATION DISORDERS (NIDOCD)
Clearing House
P.O. Box 37777
Washington, D.C. 20013-7777

1-301-496-7243
1-301-402-0252 TDD
Fax 1-301-402-0018

Publications

A Decade of Progress Ahead: Annual Report of the National Deafness and Other Communications Disorders, The 1990 annual report that describes research in taste disorders.

Smell and Taste Disorders, an 8-page booklet describing common taste problems and current research.

TAY-SACHS AND ALLIED DISEASES

Tay-Sachs disease is characterized by very early onset, progressive retardation in development, paralysis, dementia, blindness, and death by the age of 3 or 4 years. This inherited disorder is most common in families of Eastern European Jewish origin and is caused by a deficiency of an enzyme.

NATIONAL TAY-SACHS & ALLIED DISEASES, INC. (NTSAD)
2001 Beacon St.
Brookline, MA 02146

1-617-277-4463
Fax 1-617-277-0314

Purpose NTSAD is a nonprofit, voluntary health organization committed to the eradication of Tay-Sachs and related genetic diseases. Services include carrier screening, public and professional education, family services, laboratory quality control, parent support network, and research. Referrals are made to testing centers, physicians, and support groups. NTSAD also maintains an extensive lending library as well as videotapes and audiovideo material for individual and/or community use.

Publications

Child Care Manual.

Family Service.

Overview Publications on Tay-Sachs and Allied Diseases (four different pieces).

Prevent a Tragedy: Testing Center Directory.

Tay-Sachs: The Dreaded Inheritance.

Understanding Lysosomal Storage Disease.

Literature also available in Russian.

TEENAGERS

This is the period when children are in adult bodies. Many of the problems of adolescence stem from the changes in the type and pattern of their hormones. During the teen years there are physical, mental and emotional pressures that can make adolescence a difficult time for both those going through it and their parents.

COMMUNICABLE DISEASE CENTER *1-301-436-8500*

Centers for Disease Control
Scientific and Technical Information Branch
6525 Belcrest Road, Room 1064
Hyattsville, MD 20782

Publications

Office Visits by Adolescents, report of health care for adolescents ages 11 to 20.

NATIONAL INSTITUTE OF MENTAL HEALTH (NIMH) *1-301-443-2403*

Information Resources and Inquiries Branch
Office of Scientific Information, Room 15C
5900 Fishers Lane, Room 15-105
Rockville, MD 20857

Publications

Plain Talk About Adolescence, ADM 85-1065, 2 pages.

What to Do When a Friend Is Depressed: A Guide for Teenagers, OM 00 4036, 8 pages.

TEETH

The first part of your digestive system is the mouth where teeth serve the purposes of tearing and mashing the food into small pieces so that it may start its journey through your body. Teeth start out alive. The pulp at the heart of each tooth contains blood vessels and nerves that sense heat, cold, pressure and pain. Teeth hurt when they first push their way into the mouth through the gums. Then they may not be in perfect alignment and eventually they may be broken or decayed if they are not protected by proper preventive care or are subjected to trauma.

AMERICAN ACADEMY OF PERIODONTOLOGY *1-312-787-5518*
737 North Michigan Ave., Suite 800
Chicago, IL 60611-2690

Purpose The American Academy of Periodontology is a 6,200-member association of dental professionals specializing in the prevention, diagnosis, and treatment of diseases affecting the gums and supporting structures of the teeth. The Academy serves as an educational resource for periodontists and general dentists and is committed to increasing the public's awareness of periodontal disease and how it can be prevented and treated. It will refer callers to periodontists in their locale.

Publications

To obtain single copies of any brochure, send a stamped, self-addressed, business-size envelope to the above address, Attention Dept. PH. Indicate on the outer envelope which brochure(s) you are requesting.

Dental Implants: Are They Right for You? a brochure designed for the patient considering dental implants; illustrates different types of dental implants and explains how implants are used to correct a variety of dental problems.

Gum Disease: Be Tested to See If You Have It, a brochure that stresses early detection and treatment, describes how gum disease progresses, and explains what is included in a thorough periodontal exam.

Gum Disease: What You Need to Know, a brochure that serves as a guide to the causes, treatment, and prevention of periodontal disease. Also available in Spanish.

How to Brush and Floss, a brochure that provides easy-to-follow instructions on brushing and flossing and stresses the importance of regular dental visits.

Keeping Your Gums Healthy, a brochure designed for the patient who has completed the active phase of periodontal treatment; it answers some of the most frequently asked questions about maintenance therapy.

Periodontal Surgery: What Can I Expect? a brochure that explains when periodontal surgery may be needed, when to return to the periodontist, and what methods can be used to prevent the recurrence of the disease.

HEALTH AND HUMAN SERVICES, DEPARTMENT OF; PUBLIC HEALTH SERVICE; NATIONAL INSTITUTES OF HEALTH; NATIONAL INSTITUTE OF DENTAL RESEARCH; *1-301-496-4261*

Public Inquiries and Reports Section
National Institute of Dental Research
National Institute of Health
Building 31, Room 2C35
Bethesda, MD 20892

Purpose The Institute conducts research and related training on dental caries; periodontal diseases, congenital craniofacial malformations, soft tissue diseases, craniofacial pain and sensory-motor dysfunction, salivary glands and secretions, mineralized tissues and fluoride studies, pulp biology, nutrition research, behavioral studies, implants, replants, transplants, and restorative materials. The Institute maintains a data bank on its research and training grants and awards and answers callers inquiries.

Publications
A list of publications is available.

NATIONAL INSTITUTE OF DENTAL RESEARCH (NIDR) *1-301-496-4261*

Building 31, Room 2C35
Bethesda, MD 20892

Publications

Dental Tips for Diabetics. (Also available in Spanish).

Dry Mouth (Xerostomia).

Fluoride Mouthrinsing in Schools... Protection for Children's Teeth, NIH Pub. No. 82-1131.

Fluoride to Protect the Teeth of Adults, NIH Pub. No. 87-2329.

A Healthy Mouth for You and Your Baby, NIH Pub. No. 86-1255.

A Healthy Start... Fluoride Tablets for Children in Preschool Programs, NIH Pub. No. 82-1838.

Periodontal Disease and Diabetes—A Guide for Patients.

Periodontal (Gum) Disease.

Plaque: What It Is and How to Get Rid of It.

Prevent Baby Bottle Tooth Decay.

Seal Out Dental Decay, an explanation of the dental sealants available for covering the chewing surfaces of the molars.

Tooth Decay. (Also available in Spanish).

THALASSEMIA

See under Cooley's Anemia *and under* Genetic Counseling.

THYROID

The thyroid gland is a butterfly shaped gland in the neck, covering both sides and front of the windpipe. It is a "governor" of metabolism, regulator of the rate at which body fires burn. If the thyroid produces too little thyroid hormone, the heartbeat may be slowed and the person feels tired, depressed, and run down. It is estimated that there may be 6 to 7 million Americans who are hypothyroid. If there is too much thyroid hormone, the person may experience a fast, pounding heartbeat, even at rest. Other symptoms may include weight loss, muscle weakness, and fine tremors of the fingers and tongue.

THYROID FOUNDATION OF AMERICA, INC.
630 Ambulatory Care Center
Massachusetts General Hospital
Boston, MA 02114

Publication
Thyroid Disease, an 11-page booklet about hypothyroidism and hyperthyroidism.
For referral to a thyroid specialist in your area, contact:

AMERICAN THYROID ASSOCIATION
Endocrine-Metabolic Service 7D
Walter Reed Army Medical Center
Washington, D.C. 20307

TINNITUS

See also Ear

Derived from the Latin meaning "to tinkle" or "ring like a bell," it is a subjective experience where one hears a sound when no external physical sound is present. Sometimes called "head noises" or "ear ringing." Problems ranging in severity from wax pressing on the eardrum to tumors can cause tinnitus.

AMERICAN TINNITUS ASSOCIATION *1-503-248-9985*
P.O. Box 5
Portland, OR 97207

Purpose The Association carries on and supports research and educational activities relating to the treatment of tinnitus and other defects or diseases of the ear. Referrals are made to hearing professionals and to self-help networks nationwide. Public forum meetings are held with question and answer sessions and educational seminars for hearing professionals.

Publication
The American Tinnitus Association

TMJ (TEMPOROMANDIBULAR JOINT DISORDER)

This disorder occurs when the temporomandibular joint or jaw bone hinge doesn't open and close properly, which may cause ear or facial pain on chewing, talking, or swallowing. The TMJ is one of the most frequently used of all joints of the body.

AMERICAN ACADEMY OF OTOLARYNGOLOGY HEAD AND NECK SURGERY (AAOHNS)
One Prince Street
Alexandria, VA 22314
1-703-836-4444
Fax 1-703-683-5100

Publication
Send a stamped, self-addressed envelope for *Pain and the TMJ.*

TORSION DYSTONIA

Torsion dystonia is a rare, progressive syndrome, usually beginning in childhood and involving bizarre postures. The disorder is progressive, and in advanced stages, the person is twisted into fixed postures like a pretzel. The cause is little understood, although some believe it is genetic.

NATIONAL INSTITUTE OF NEUROLOGICAL DISORDERS AND STROKE (NINDS)
Building 31, Room 8A06
Bethesda, MD 20892
1-301-496-5751

Publication
Torsion Dystonia, NIH Pub. No. 82-717.

TORTICOLLIS

Spasmodic torticollis (ST) is a neurological disorder that affects the muscles of the neck, causing the head to pull, turn, or jerk toward the shoulder. Usually chronic, it can begin at any time in life. About 3 out of every 10,000 persons are affected. Although caused by a dysfunction in the brain, its symptoms are limited to sustained or intermittent involuntary contractions of the muscles around the neck which control the position of the head.

NATIONAL SPASMODIC TORTICOLLIS ASSOCIATION *1-800-HURTFUL*
P.O. 476
Elm Grove, WI 53122

Purpose The Association provides support and information for people afflicted with torticollis and refers callers to support groups and physicians who treat the condition.

Publication

Spasmodic Torticollis: What Is It? What Are the Symptoms? Is Help Available? a brochure.

TOURETTE SYNDROME (TS)

It begins in childhood with simple tics but progresses to multiple jerks and vocal tics. The latter may begin as grunting or barking noises and evolve into compulsive utterances.

NATIONAL INSTITUTE OF NEUROLOGICAL DISORDERS AND STROKE (NINDS) *1-301-496-5751*
Building 31, Room 8A06
Bethesda, MD 20892

Publication

Tourette Syndrome, NIH Pub. No. 83-2163.

TOURETTE SYNDROME ASSOCIATION (TSA) *1-718-224-2999*
42-40 Bell Blvd. *1-800-237-0717*
Bayside, NY 11361

Purpose TSA and its 44 chapters are involved in educating the public and professional communities about TS. Chapters provide inservice programs locally. TSA chapters will make referrals to physicians and self-help groups.

Publications

Newsletter and TSA publication list.

TOXOPLASMOSIS

Toxoplasmosis is a disease caused by a small parasite that can infect any warmblooded animal, including humans. It may cause no symptoms in adults but can cause miscarriage or stillbirth when pregnant women are infected.

NATIONAL INSTITUTE OF ALLERGY AND INFECTIOUS DISEASES *1-301-496-5717*
Building 31, Room 7A32
Bethesda, MD 20892

Publication

Toxoplasmosis, NIH Pub. No. 83-308.

TRANQUILIZERS

See Aging.

TRANSPLANTATION

See also under Kidney.

The success rates of transplant surgery continue to improve. Unfortunately, the availability of transplants to those who need them is limited by growing shortages in the supply of organs and tissues donated. At this writing, 22,000 patients were listed on a national waiting list for organ transplants. Many are doomed to die because no transplant organs will be available for them.

Vital organs may be procured and transported thousands of miles to a recipient center for transplantation. This is due, in part, to advances in preservation techniques.

DOW CHEMICAL COMPANY'S TAKE INITIATIVE
PROGRAM ON TRANSPLANTATION
500 N. Michigan Ave.
Chicago, IL 60611

Publication

Transplant a Miracle, answers the most commonly asked questions about organ donation and transplantation—what organs can be donated, who can become a donor, religious positions on the issue, and more.

NATIONAL CENTER FOR RESEARCH RESOURCES (NCRR) *1-301-496-5545*
Westwood Building, Room 857
Bethesda, MD 20892

Publications

Facts About Heart and Heart/Lung Transplant, NIH Pub. No. 90-2990.
Research Advances in Human Transplantation.

NATIONAL KIDNEY FOUNDATION, INC. *1-800-622-9010*
30 East 33rd St.
New York, NY 10016

TRAUMA

See American Trauma Society *under* Emergencies.

TRAVEL

Being sick is bad enough but to be ill away from home is disastrous, especially if you do not speak the local language. A sore ear or an upset stomach may be magnified when you don't know the qualifications of the available doctor, and a serious problem such as a heart attack or an injury can be life threatening. Preparation in advance about access to prescreened physicians who speak English is always wise, even if you are strong and healthy before you leave. It is the same principle as taking out insurance for an event that may never occur.

INTERNATIONAL ASSOCIATION FOR MEDICAL
ASSISTANCE TO TRAVELLERS (IAMAT) *1-716-754-4883*
417 Center Street
Lewiston, NY 14092

Purpose Established in 1960, IAMAT is a voluntary organization of hospitals, health care centers, and physicians throughout the world who pledge to provide travelers in distress with physicians who speak their language; who meet IAMAT's standards, which are generally consistent with American standards; and who adhere to a fixed fee schedule. The Association provides information on malaria risk, immunization requirements, schistosomiasis risk, Chagas' disease risk; sanitary conditions of water, milk, and food; and climatic conditions. Refers to physicians in about 500 cities in 120 countries (excluding United States). Membership is free; however, donations are appreciated to continue research and climate charts are only given to donors.

Publications

Be Aware of Schistosomiasis.
How to Protect Yourself Against Malaria.
Traveller Clinical Record.
24 World Climate Charts.
When Hiking in Latin America Be Alert to Chagas' Disease.
World Immunization Chart.
World Malaria Risk Chart.
World Schistosomiasis Risk Chart.

TREMOR

Tremor is a common symptom of neurologic disease and may be due to trauma, tumor, stroke, or degenerative disease. The most common tremor condition is idiopathic or essential (cause unknown) or hereditary tremor. In fact, essential tremor is the most common of all neurologic conditions. It is estimated that 3 to 4 million people in the United States alone have such tremor. In over half the cases the disease runs in families. The condition is transmitted as an autosomal dominant inheritance, which means that the offspring of an affected individual will have a 50 percent chance of also having the illness.

The tremor can start in adolescence or adulthood. Both genders are equally affected. The mean age at onset is 45 years. When tremor begins in the very elderly, it has sometimes been called senile tremor. The condition is slowly progressive, and tremors will worsen over time. Some individuals may have to change occupations (i.e., dentists, draftsmen) or have to take early retirement.

Tremor may involve different body parts. Most often the hands are affected. Usually the dominant hand is first affected and eventually both hands may be involved. Handwriting becomes less legible, and drinking liquids is difficult to manage. The individual may have to use both hands or use a straw to drink. Eating soup may become impossible. Dysfunction with fine manipulation and embarrassment are also problems. Tremor of the head may also occur. The shakiness may be a "yes-yes" or a "no-no" movement. Embarrassment and social withdrawal may result from head tremor. Shakiness of the voice may occur, which gives a quavering intonation to speaking. Tremor of the trunk and legs is seen in some patients.

Tremor is the sole symptom of this disorder, and other neurologic problems rarely occur. Stress and social interaction usually worsen the tremor. It may no longer be possible to sign a check in a bank or serve coffee at a luncheon. Small amounts of alcohol may temporarily relieve the tremor, but the use of large amounts of alcohol may be harmful. Unfortunately, the tremor is not often recognized by physicians who may misdiagnose it as anxiety or Parkinson's disease. There is also the misbelief that nothing medically can be done to relieve the tremor.

Little is known about what causes this tremor; hence the eponym essential or idiopathic, which means that the cause is unknown, as with essential hypertension. Essential tremor is certainly a disorder of the central nervous system. However, it is not known what area of the brain is involved. It is also unclear why the disease occurs and how it affects the brain. A better understanding of these mechanisms would lead to better treatment and/or preventive therapy.

INTERNATIONAL TREMOR FOUNDATION (ITF) *1-312-664-2344*
360 West Superior Street
Chicago, IL 60610

Purpose The International Tremor Foundation is a nonprofit organization which derives its support entirely from its membership and the general public. A large portion of operating expenses is allocated to patient and family services. The office in Chicago is maintained so that members may call or write for a personal response to specific questions. A Medical Advisory Board is accessible for consultation to the staff on such matters and to supervise publication content and preparation. The office staff is establishing an extensive referral service to guide patients and families to proper clinical care.

The ITF has a program of educational symposia for patients and families. These take the format of experts in the field of tremor research and clinical care addressing lay audiences in various cities around the United States. These symposia consist of presentations by physicians followed by a question and answer session.

Publications
Newsletters, written primarily for patient and family educational reporting in layperson's language. The newsletters, which are published four times each year, report on recent advances in research, answer questions of general interest to members, and publish members' suggestions. Additionally, space is offered to other groups which provide emotional support and social opportunities for patients and their families.

TUBEROUS SCLEROSIS (TS)

Tuberous sclerosis is a multifaceted genetic disease characterized by growths in the skin, viscera, and/or skeleton, producing a variety of symptoms, including seizures, mental retardation, skin and eye abnormalities, and behavior problems.

NATIONAL INSTITUTE OF NEUROLOGICAL DISORDERS AND STROKE (NINDS) *1-301-496-5751*
Building 31, Room 8A06
Bethesda, MD 20892

Publication
Tuberous Sclerosis, NIH Pub. No. 85-1846.

NATIONAL TUBEROUS SCLEROSIS ASSOCIATION (NTSA) *1-301-459-9888*
8000 Corporate Drive, Suite 120 *1-800-225-6872*
Landover, MD 20785

Purpose NTSA seeks to improve the quality of life for individuals and families affected by tuberous sclerosis through

- The encouragement and support of research into the diagnosis, cause, management, and cure of tuberous sclerosis.
- The development of a national network for family support and the education of medical and allied professionals. It does not refer to physicians, but it does have a national support network of parents and other people affected by tuberous sclerosis.

A network of state representatives has been established nationwide to promote group meetings and telephone referral between families. Offers genetic counseling; genetic markers. Answers inquiries; provides advisory and reference services; conducts seminars and workshops; distributes publications; makes referrals to other sources of information; operates speakers' bureau. Services are free and available to anyone.

Publications
Fact sheets, parent brochures, physician's brochures, other articles, papers and information on tuberous sclerosis.

TURNER'S SYNDROME

This chromosomal abnormality affects 1 in every 2,500 girls born each year. It is caused by the absence of, or a structural defect in, one of the X chromosomes in the cells. Short stature is the most visible characteristic of Turner's syndrome: the average height of a woman with Turner's is 4 feet 8 inches. Most women with the syndrome do not have ovaries. Since ovaries normally produce estrogen, Turner's women lack this essential hormone. This results in infertility and incomplete sexual development—the two other major characteristics of this syndrome.

TURNER'S SYNDROME SOCIETY
7777 Kelle St., Floor 3
Concord, Ontario L4K 1Y7
Canada

Purpose Partially supported by Health and Welfare Canada, Ontario Department of Health, and Ontario Department of Community and Social Services, the Society offers support to individuals with Turner's syndrome and their families and seeks to educate the public about Turner's syndrome, genetic disorders, gonadal dysgenesis, short stature, and secondary sex characteristics. The Society will answer questions and will refer to self-help groups.

Publications

Quarterly newsletter.

Video documentary.

The X's and O's of Turner's Syndrome, a comprehensive, up-to-date information 39-page booklet.

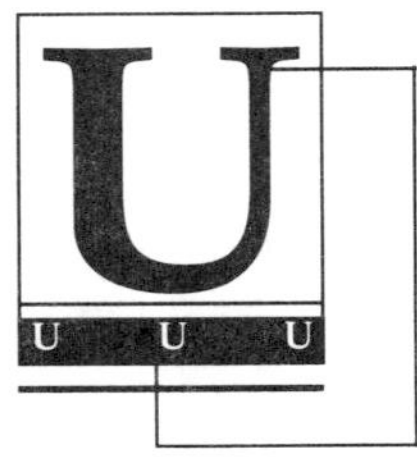

ULCERATIVE COLITIS AND CROHN'S DISEASE

See also Digestive Diseases.

Ulcerative colitis is a chronic condition in which raw, inflamed areas called culers and small abscesses develop in the lining of the large intestine. Symptoms usually recur over a period of years. A characteristic early symptom is left-sided abdominal pain that is relieved by a bowel movement. In a severe attack, there may be painful bowel movements, sweating, nausea, loss of appetite, and a high fever.

NATIONAL INSTITUTES OF HEALTH (NIH) *1-301-496-2563*
Office of Clinical Center Communications
Building 10, Room 1C255
Bethesda, MD 20892

Publication

Ulcerative Colitis and Crohn's Disease, a videotape that can be borrowed.

ULCERS

An ulcer is a defect in the tissue lining of the digestive tract. Duodenal ulcers are located in the part of the small intestines connected to the stomach (the duodenum). They are about four times more common than gastric ulcers, which are those occurring in the stomach lining. The term "peptic ulcer" includes ulcers in both sites. An ulcer is an open sore on any external or internal surface of the body. Peptic ulcer disease is one of the more common digestive diseases. Between 10 percent and 20 percent of Americans are thought to suffer from it at some time during their lives.

NATIONAL INSTITUTE OF DIABETES AND DIGESTIVE AND KIDNEY DISEASES (NIDDKD) *1-301-499-3583*
Building 31, Room 9A04
Bethesda, MD 20892

Publication

About Stomach Ulcers, NIH Pub. No. 87-676.

URINARY INCONTINENCE

Urinary incontinence is very common among older Americans and is epidemic in nursing homes, according to the Simon Foundation. It costs Americans more than $10 billion each year and leads to stigmatization and social isolation. Urinary incontinence is not part of normal aging, but age-related changes predispose to its occurrence.

HELP FOR INCONTINENT PEOPLE, INC. (HIP) *1-803-579-7900*
P.O. Box 544 *1-800-BLADDER*
Union, SC 29379

Purpose HIP is a nonprofit organization dedicated to improving the quality of life for people who are incontinent. HIP is a source of education, advocacy, and support to the public and to the health profession about the causes, prevention, diagnosis, treatments, and management alternatives for incontinence. Referrals are made to physicians who specialize in the diagnosis and treatment of incontinence.

Publications

For Your Information, an information sheet about the services supplied by HIP and a list of publications for sale.

The HIP Report, a quarterly newsletter that contains easy-to-read articles by doctors and nurses about the causes and treatments of incontinence. Members share successful methods for curing or managing their bladder control problems. Advertisers show their latest products, and there are always valuable discount coupons.

NATIONAL INSTITUTE ON AGING (NIA)
Public Inquiries
Federal Building, Room 6C12
Bethesda, MD 20892

SIMON FOUNDATION *1-708-864-3913*
P.O. Box 835 *1-800-23SIMON*
Wilmette, IL 60091

Purpose The Foundation's mission is to bring the topic of incontinence out of the closet, remove the stigma, and provide help and education to those suffering from incontinence, their families, and the health professionals who provide their care. Referrals are made to a nationwide network of "I WILL Manage" education/support groups and to health care professionals.

Publications

A free information packet is available which elaborates the Foundation's services and includes a copy of the *Informer*, a quarterly newsletter.

Urinary Incontinence.

URINARY TRACT PROBLEMS

The urinary tract consists of the kidneys, the ureter, and the urethra. The kidneys, which look like large kidney beans, are behind the intestines and just above the waist on either side of the spine. Each kidney contains over 1 million tiny filters called glomeruli, which remove waste and excess water from the blood to form urine. A narrow muscular tube, the ureter, carries the urine from each kidney down to the bladder, a temporary storage place in the lower abdomen. Periodically, the contents of the bladder passes out of the body through another tube, the urethra.

The usual symptoms of urinary tract infections include burning, pain and/or discomfort in the bladder area, intense urge to urinate, fever, chills, and lower abdominal pain. A UTI is more common in women than in men, due to the configuration of the female system. A UTI is caused when bacteria enter the body through the urethra, the tube that carries urine out from the bladder to be excreted. The female urethra is only about 1 inch long compared to a considerably longer urethra in men. Women are also more susceptible to UTI because the external openings of the urethra, vagina, and the intestinal tract are in such close proximity that bacteria can move easily from one to the other. In men, a UTI is usually the sign of a specific anatomical abnormality such as an enlarged prostate or retaining large amounts of urine in the bladder after urination.

NATIONAL INSTITUTE OF DIABETES AND DIGESTIVE AND KIDNEY DISEASES (NIDDKD) *1-301-499-3583*
Building 31, Room 9A04
Bethesda, MD 20892
For publications, write or call:

NATIONAL KIDNEY AND UROLOGIC DISEASES INFORMATION CLEARING HOUSE *1-301-468-6345*
Box NKUDIC
9000 Rockville Pike
Bethesda, MD 20892

Publications

Use the number following the publication description as well as the name of the publication.

Extracorporeal Shock-Wave Lithotripsy, a patient and public education fact sheet. Describes the procedure for the removal of kidney and urinary tract stones. Discusses underlying principle, effectiveness, and side effects of lithotripsy. (10)

Prevention and Treatment of Kidney Stones, a patient and public education booklet. Describes etiology, symptoms, diagnosis, and treatment of kidney and urinary tract stones. (4)

Prostate Enlargement: Benign Prostatic Hyperplasia (BPH), a patient and public education brochure. Gives basic information about the prostate gland and prostate enlargement; describes symptoms, diagnosis, and treatment. (22)

Prostate Problems, a patient and public education fact sheet. Describes common prostate problems such as acute prostatitis, chronic prostatitis, and benign prostatic hypertrophy prostate cancer; surgery and prevention are outlined. National Institute on Aging. (7)

Understanding Urinary Tract Infections, a patient and public education booklet. Describes causes, symptoms, diagnosis, and treatment of urinary tract infections. (3)

Urinary Incontinence, a patient and public education fact sheet. Describes diagnosis, treatment, and types of urinary incontinence. National Institute on Aging. (6)

Urinary Incontinence in Adults. (37)

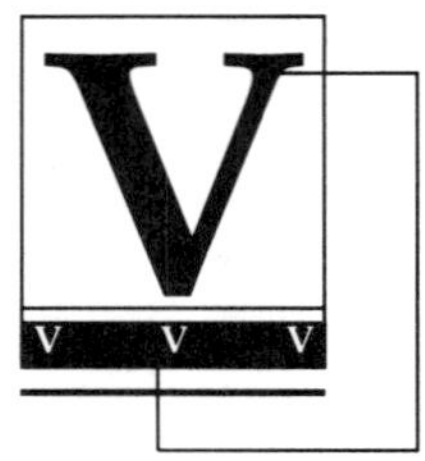

VASCULITIS

See page 30.

VERTIGO

There is a complex relationship between your inner ears and your eyes—a system that is often called the sixth sense. It involves motion, balance, acceleration, and velocity. When something goes wrong with the mechanism, the result can be dizziness, nausea, and eye difficulties.

AMERICAN ACADEMY OF OTOLARYNGOLOGY
HEAD AND NECK SURGERY (AAOHNS)
One Prince Street
Alexandria, VA 22314

Publication
Send a stamped, self-addressed envelope for
Dizziness and Motion Sickness.

NATIONAL INSTITUTE ON DEAFNESS
AND OTHER COMMUNICATION DISORDERS (NIDOCD) *1-301-496-7243*
Building 31, Room 1B62
Bethesda, MD 20892

Publication
Dizziness, NIH Pub. No. 86-76, a 27-page booklet describing causes of dizziness.

VESTIBULAR DISORDERS ASSOCIATION (VEDA)
P.O. Box 4467
Portland, OR 97208-4467

Purpose VEDA provides support groups for those suffering from vestibular (dizziness) and related disorders and makes referrals to physicians and clinics.

Publications
Booklets.
Brochures.
Fact sheets.
Quarterly newsletter.

VETERANS

See also Mental Health.

Those who served in the armed forces are entitled to many benefits. The key is knowing which benefits and whom to contact to obtain them.

PARALYZED VETERANS OF AMERICA (PVA)
Public Education and Communication Department
801 18th Street, N.W.
Washington, DC 20006

1-202-872-1300
1-800-232-1782
Veterans' Referral Line
1-202-416-7622 TDD

Purpose The Paralyzed Veterans of America was founded in 1946 as a national service organization to meet the needs of veterans who were paralyzed as a result of disease or an injury to the spinal cord. The PVA is supported by donations from the general public. It works to ensure quality health care and rehabilitation and civil rights for veterans with spinal cord injuries and all persons with a disability. PVA supports legislation and advances in medicine and technology through various programs, activities, and departments such as the Spinal Cord Research Foundation, a Medical Affairs Program, The Education and Training Foundation, a national research program, the National Advocacy Program; a national legislation program, the National Service Program, and the National Sports and Recreation Program. PVA's Veterans Benefits Department's primary mission is to ensure that those who are entitled have access to all appropriate Department of Veterans Affairs (VA) resources and federal and state benefits. PVA's Veterans Benefits Department provides benefits counseling and claims assistance via a PVAA-funded service network of 59 service offices located in VA facilities nationwide. These services are open to all veterans, their dependents, and beneficiaries.

Publications
Serving The Veteran, an informational brochure.

VIDEO DISPLAY TERMINALS (VDTs)

Video display terminals are a staple in today's workplace. The most common complaints from constant VDT users are dry or burning eyes, eye fatigue, blurred vision, and aches in the neck and back, according to the Federal Drug Administration. Here are some hints to prevent discomfort:

1. Use good room lighting. The typical office lighting may be too bright for computer work.
2. Eliminate sources of glare. Don't sit facing a bright window.
3. Adjust screen brightness and contrast.
4. Take a 15-minute break every hour from highly demanding computer tasks and don't forget to blink frequently to reduce dryness and look at distant objects to relax your eyes.
5. Maintain a good viewing distance. Close viewing may cause focusing fatigue. Adjust workstations so that keyboard, screen, and paper copy are equal distance from the eyes with the screen slightly below eye level.
6. Keep work environment free of dust.

AMERICAN PHYSICAL THERAPY ASSOCIATION
1111 North Fairfax St.
Alexandria, VA 22314

Publications
Send a stamped, self-addressed envelope for
Carpal Tunnel Syndrome.
Posture and Back Problems Related to VDTs.

OCCUPATIONAL SAFETY AND HEALTH ADMINISTRATION *1-202-523-8148*
200 Constitution Ave., N.W., Room N 3101
Washington, D.C. 20210

Publication
Send a self-addressed label and request for
Working Safely with VDTs, OSHA Pub. No. 3092.

VISION

See also Blindness, Eyes.

VISION FOUNDATION, INC. *1-800-852-3929 (in Massachusetts only)*
818 Mt. Auburn St.
Watertown, MA 02172

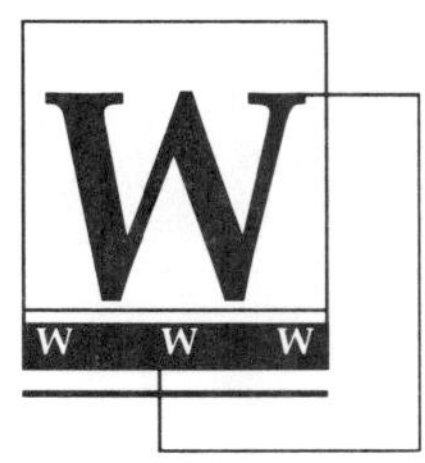

WEATHER

See under Aging.

WOMEN'S HEALTH

1-202-293-6045

The anatomical differences between men and women are obvious. It has only been recently acknowledged that women suffer many of the same ills as men, including heart attacks and cancer and yet it has been found that often their complaints about symptoms are not taken as seriously as men's.

AMERICAN COLLEGE OF OBSTETRICIANS AND GYNECOLOGISTS RESOURCE CENTER *1-202-638-5577*
409 12th Street, S.W.
Washington, D.C. 20024-2188

Purpose With a membership of more than 31,000 physicians specializing in obstetrics-gynecologic care, the College serves as a strong advocate for quality health care for women; maintaining the highest standards of clinical practice and continuing education for its members; promoting patient education and stimulating patient understanding, and involvement in, medical care; and increasing awareness among its members and the public of the changing issues facing women's health care. It responds to specific questions, and it refers to physicians and associations.

Publications

Contraception, a pamphlet that describes how the various contraceptives work.

The Pap Test, a pamphlet that explains the procedure and its value and includes a glossary.

Patient Education, an order form for the many other educational pamphlets and books provided by the College.

Premenstrual Syndrome, a pamphlet that describes a group of physical or behavioral changes that some women go through before their menstrual periods begin.

NATIONAL INSTITUTE ON AGING (NIA) *1-301-496-1752*
Federal Building, Room 6C12
Bethesda, MD 20892

Publication
Health Resources for Older Women, NIH Pub. No. 87-2899.

NATIONAL WOMEN'S HEALTH RESOURCE CENTER *1-202-293-6045*
2440 M Street, N.W., Suite 201
Washington, D.C. 20037

Purpose The Center works to enable women to heighten their knowledge and increase participation in their own health care and maintain healthy and productive lives. It promotes professional and public education and research that focuses on diseases or conditions that affect women, provides advocacy on women's health issues and disseminates information, maintains a speakers' bureau, bestows annual Breast Cancer Awareness Awards, and provides free health information and referrals to physicians and self-help groups by phone.

Publications
Newsletter, videotapes, and other publications are available for a fee.

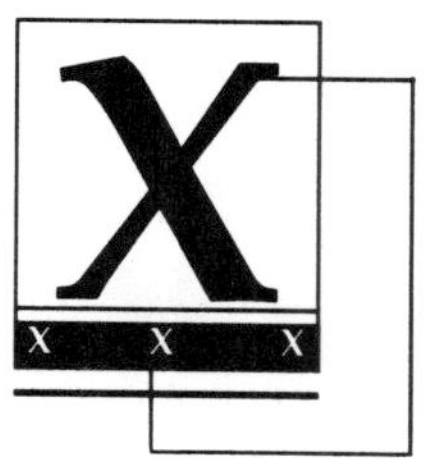

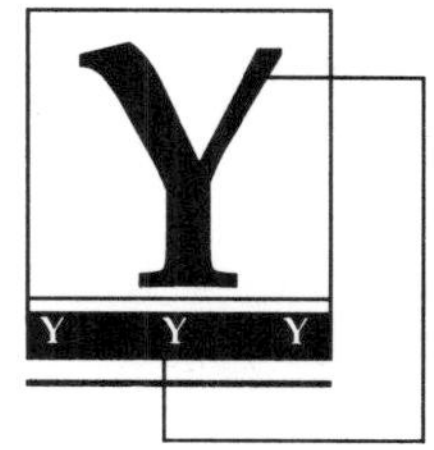

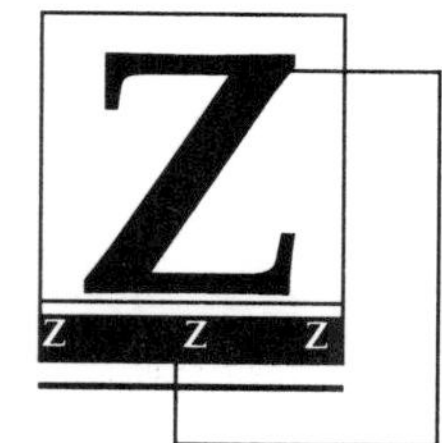

X-RAYS

AMERICAN COLLEGE OF RADIOLOGY *1-800-227-5463*
1891 Preston White Drive
Reston, VA 22091

Purpose The college seeks to advance the science of radiology, improve radiologic service to the patient, study the economic aspects of the practice of radiology, and encourage improved and continuing education for radiologists and allied professional fields.

Publications
Patient information pamphlets; booklets on radiation cancer treatments and diagnostic radiology.

AMERICAN SOCIETY FOR THERAPEUTIC RADIOLOGY ONCOLOGY (ASTRO) *1-703-648-8900*
1891 Preston White Drive
Reston, VA 22091

Purpose The Society's aims are to extend the benefits of radiation therapy to patients with cancer or other disorders, to advance its scientific basis, and to provide for the education and professional fellowship of its members.

Publications
Curing Cancer with Radiation Therapy, a booklet.

Patient information pamphlets on radiation oncology.

INDEX

A

D

E

F

G

H

I

J

K

L

M

N

O

S

T